NEUROSCIENCE RESEARCH PROGRESS

ELECTROMYOGRAPHY

NEW DEVELOPMENTS, PROCEDURES AND APPLICATIONS

NEUROSCIENCE RESEARCH PROGRESS

Additional books in this series can be found on Nova's website under the Series tab.

Additional e-books in this series can be found on Nova's website under the e-book tab.

MUSCULAR SYSTEM - ANATOMY, FUNCTIONS AND INJURIES

Additional books in this series can be found on Nova's website under the Series tab.

Additional e-books in this series can be found on Nova's website under the e-book tab.

NEUROSCIENCE RESEARCH PROGRESS

ELECTROMYOGRAPHY

NEW DEVELOPMENTS, PROCEDURES AND APPLICATIONS

HIROKI TAKADA
EDITOR

New York

For permission to use material from this book please contact us:
Telephone 631-231-7269; Fax 631-231-8175
Web Site: http://www.novapublishers.com

NOTICE TO THE READER

Library of Congress Cataloging-in-Publication Data

Library of Congress Control Number: 2012937171

ISBN: 978-1-62081-717-9

Published by Nova Science Publishers, Inc. † New York

Contents

Preface

Hiroki Takada*
University of Fukui, Fukui, Japan

Italian physician L. Galvani demonstrated the relationship between electricity and muscle contraction that occurs in the electric fluid carried to the muscles by the nerves. He coined the term *animal electricity* to describe the muscle-activating force. One hundred and fifty years after he determined that muscle activation is generated by an electric fluid carried by the nerves, mathematician N. Wiener studied an artificial hand controlled by an electrical current produced in the muscles. He proposed *cybernetics*, which focused on the myoelectric (ME) potential of approximately -90 mV, as recorded using electromyograms. The ME potential in skeletal muscles is often measured and recorded. Biosignals are generated by the following mechanisms:

1) Form: Both ends of the skeletal muscles are adhered to the bones by tendons. Muscle fibers are 50–100 μm in diameter and are aligned longitudinally in a muscle cell. The fibers consist of muscular fibrils that are 1–2 μm in diameter and contain 2 types of filaments (*Chapter 11*). A sarcomere is the morphological unit of a muscle fiber, which is located between disc-like Z bands that partition the fibrils into 2 portions.
2) Route: The (efferent) nerve impulse (action potential) from the primary motor cortex (M1) cooperates with the premotor area and is transferred to α-motor neurons in the spinal cord through the pyramidal tracts, extrapyramidal tracts, and brainstem. It arrives at the motor end plate through the terminal axon and results in muscle cell membrane excitation. This excitation transforms both sides of the muscle fiber. The membrane current is generated by depolarization of the muscle membrane. Changes in electrical potential (7–20 Hz) occur in the membrane current through the surrounding volume conductor. Muscular motion follows the abovementioned biosignal process (*Chapters 1 and 11*).

ME potentials are induced by changes in nerve impulse firing patterns. Muscle fibers that are controlled by a motor nerve are collectively called a motor unit (MU), several of which can be excited by nerve impulses, producing an MU action potential. The MU action potential

* takada@u-fukui.ac.jp.

measured on the skin surface is the surface ME potential and is observed at a site that is spatially distant from the site at which MU action potential waves are generated. Larger MUs possess faster contraction speeds and fatigue accumulation. Electromyography (EMG) is used to detect an anomalous MU in the clinical setting.

EMG is a technique used for evaluating and recording electrical activity in the muscles, which aids in the diagnosis of neuromuscular diseases such as neuropathy, carpal tunnel syndrome, pinched nerves, herniated discs, peripheral nerve damage, and amyotrophic lateral sclerosis. Several electromyographic methods are currently used, but needle EMG (nEMG) and surface EMG (sEMG) are most often applied in the clinical setting (*Chapters 1, 2, 3, and 4*). To physiologically evaluate the electromyographic wave patterns for detecting abnormalities, wave patterns obtained using nEMG or sEMG are macroscopically examined and subjectively judged by physicians. *Chapters 4 and 5* introduce EMG analytical methods. After these chapters, we discuss new studies on sEMG for facial muscles (*Chapters 6 and 7*), masticatory/swallowing muscles (*Chapter 8*). Simultaneous EMG measurements are described in *Chapters 8 and 9.* Processes of human motion and behavior are evaluated by EMG (Chapters *8, 9, and 10).*

In: Electromyography
Editor: Hiroki Takada
ISBN: 978-1- 62081-717-9

Chapter I

Surface Electromyography and Its Use in Clinical Applications

Usha Kuruganti and Victoria Chester
University of New Brunswick, Fredericton,
New Brunswick, Canada

Abstract

Human movement is a complex process and as the number of movements increase, the processes involved become even more complicated. Understanding how voluntary movements are generated and the methods used to measure them can help our understanding of human performance. One method of monitoring muscle behaviour is surface electromyography (sEMG). The properties of muscle allow its electrical activity to be recorded under different states. sEMG employs the use of electrodes placed over the skin of the muscle(s) of interest to detect and record this electrical activity. Various mathematical techniques are then used to process the data. The information in the recorded signal provides significant information including an indication of muscle activity, temporal parameters (i.e. how long the muscle is activated and when it turns on and off), an estimate of the force produced, indications of fatigue and muscle co-contraction (simultaneous activity of agonist and antagonist muscles). The interpretation of sEMG becomes more complex when examining data from clinical populations due to a number of factors such as modifications in muscle architecture and the nature of the disease or disorder. This chapter will discuss current techniques used to collect sEMG from clinical populations, methods to analyze the data and the current challenges faced when applying this technique to clinical groups. Areas for future research will also be addressed.

Introduction

Surface electromyography (sEMG) is a useful diagnostic tool for clinicians. This technique has been used for a wide array of purposes. The advent of different types of systems, including wireless systems, has increased the use of sEMG with clinical groups. While the ease of which data can be recorded has improved greatly over the years, care must be taken with applying this technique to clinical populations, particularly since depending on the disease or disorder there may be significant physiological and biomechanical alterations in the patient. In spite of these concerns, sEMG remains a useful tool for understanding muscle activation patterns of those with affected musculature.

Physiology of Muscle Contraction

Voluntary contractions are those motions about which we are consciously aware. We use voluntary contractions every day when we pick up a book, open a jar or turn a key. The sequence of events to lift a book, for example, is very complex. First, one needs to use senses (e.g. sight) to locate the book and then compute a trajectory to actually reach out and locate the book in space. Then, one needs to calculate how far to open and close the hand to grasp the book and compute the amount of force needed.

Voluntary movement is a complex process involving both neural and muscular activity. This complex process is known as the cross-bridge theory of muscle contraction and is described in detail elsewhere (Huxley, 2000, 1957).Briefly, muscles respond to the central nervous system (CNS) commands by sending information regarding the muscle back to the CNS through sensory (afferent) neurons to the brain where the information is processed. The brain makes adjustments to the original message and then sends out further messages to the muscle through the efferent motor neurons to adjust the movement. This process continues for the duration of the desired activity. The many physiological processes that occur during muscle contraction including the depolarization and repolarization of the membrane at the neuromuscular junction, result in electrical activity of the muscles. In order to sustain a muscle contraction, the motor units (MUs) must be repeatedly activated, and this sequence is called a motor unit action potential train (MUAPT). The summation of action potentials from the homogeneous muscle fibers of a motor unit form the typical biphasic or triphasic waveshape of a single motor unit action potential (MUAP). Electromyography (EMG) is used to measure the sum of the action potentials and reflects the electrical activity that results from muscle contraction (Figure 1).

Surface Electromyography Measurement

Surface electromyography (sEMG) is the measurement of the electrical activity, (i.e. muscle action potentials) at the skin's surface, that brings about muscle contraction. The sum of action potentials can be detected at the muscle surface using electrodes placed over the belly of the muscle. The recorded signal or the sEMG consists of the weighted sum of the electrical contributions of active MUs and contains information about the characteristics and physiology of the active MUs (Karlsson et al., 2009). The shape of each MUAP depends on the number and anatomical characteristics of the innervated muscle fibers, and on the properties of the recording electrodes (Farina et al., 2002b).

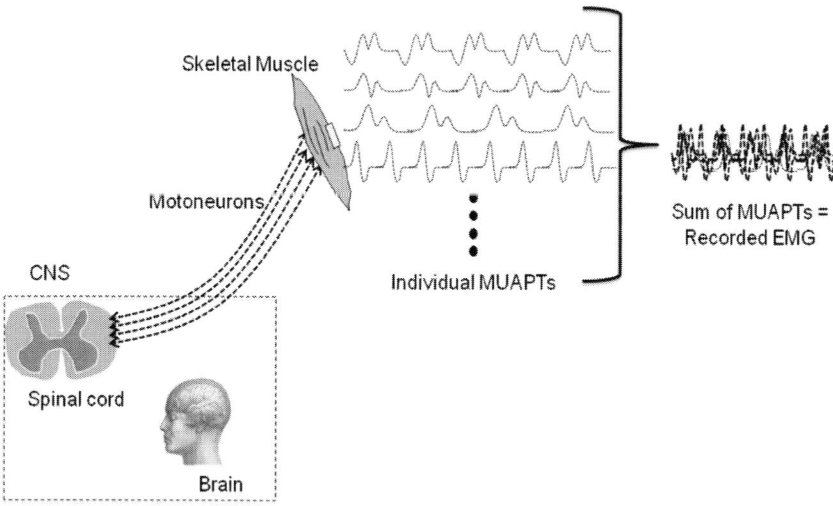

Figure 1. Simplified overview of several MUAPTs and the resulting EMG that is recorded at the surface of the skin.

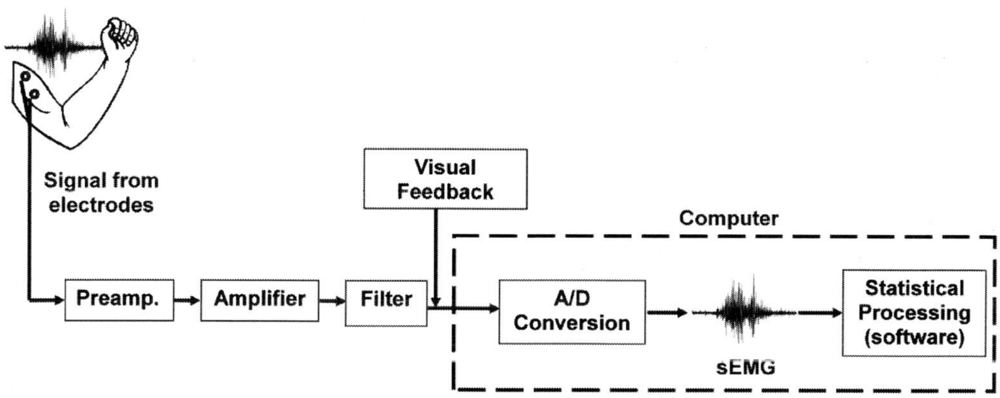

Figure 2. Surface EMG Detection. Overview of the use of surface electrodes to record the signal resulting from muscle contraction.

It has been shown that under static conditions, the sEMG is related to force production and can be used to better understand activation (DeLuca, 1997; Basmajian&DeLuca, 1985; Karlsson et al., 2009). The amplitude of the signal relates to the force required and is reflective of motor unit recruitment where more and more motor units are activated and their frequency of firing increases, increasing the force. The typical range of the amplitude of the EMG is 0.01 – 5 mV. The frequency content of the signal ranges between 1 and 3000 Hz for surface electrodes, however it is rarely over 500 Hz in practice The EMG amplitude is affected by a number of factors including the number and size of muscle fibers, the size and orientation of the electrode detection surface, the distance between the active fibers and the detection electrodes.

In order to record the EMG data, surface electrodes are placed over the muscle of interest and, in order to increase the amplitude of the signal, the data detected is fed into a series of preamplifiers and amplifiers. The signal may then be filtered in order to remove any unwanted noise. Finally, the signal is converted from analog to digital for further viewing and analysis (Figure 2).

The method used to collect EMG data is well established and is straightforward for clinical use. However, care must be taken due to the inherent instability of the signal. The sEMG can be affected by noise sources including electronic components, ambient noise, and motion artefact due to the electrode skin interface as well as physiological factors including injury or disease of the muscle.

The sEMG assumes that the recorded electric potentials originate from the muscle directly under the electrodes, however potentials from other muscles may also reach the recording site and contribute to the recorded signal (DeLuca, 1997; Disselhorst-Klug et al., 2009). This phenomenon is referred to as muscle 'crosstalk.' Crosstalk can be reduced with a variety of techniques including proper placement of the electrodes (Criswell, 2011), and adapted filter techniques (Merletti& Parker, 2004), however it cannot be avoided. Crosstalk is the main risk in the clinical use of sEMG, because most of the clinically relevant information is related to the on/off of the muscle activity that is altered by crosstalk (Merlo &Campanini, 2010). Further, the measurement of motor action potentials using EMG does not provide information on muscle tension or the contribution of passive stretch to muscle tension (Sutherland, 2001).

Applications of sEMG

The amplitude of the sEMG is often used to estimate the magnitude of the neural activation sent to muscle (through associating its amplitude with the number of action potentials discharged by a group of motor neurons), however there are some limitations to this theory (Farina et al., 2010). One limitation is that the size of a MUAP at the skin's surface is only partly related to motor neuron size (Farina et al., 2010). Secondly, the contribution of an action potential to the amplitude of the sEMG may differ across conditions (Dimitrova&Dimitrova, 2003). It has been suggested that an alternative is to use individual MU action potential discharge times (occurrence times) to estimate motor output from the spinal cord. This method, however, is currently limited to isometric, low force contractions and complete decoding of neural drive likely requires data both from surface and indwelling electrodes (Farina et al., 2010).

The sEMG can be used to examine muscle activation patterns for a variety of applications. Understanding the muscles that are activated during movement provides significant information regarding coordination. The sEMG has had many uses in clinical applications. Therapeutic uses of sEMG include the assessment of kinesiology and disorders of motor control (Pullman et al., 2000). However sEMG has not been shown to be the preferred method in certain types of assessment. For example, sEMG is significantly inferior to needle EMG for the evaluation of patients with neuromuscular disorders (Pullman et al., 2000). The sEMG has been used to examine the association between low back pain and muscle fatigue with limited success (Lehman, 2002, Pullman et al., 2000). The sEMG recorded from residual limbs of amputees have been used for many years for myoelectric control of powered prostheses (Parker et al., 2006). Parameters of the sEMG have also provided clinicians with an understanding of the muscle mechanics involved in movement.

The ability to determine if a particular muscle is activated (or not) during a movement provides clinicians with significant information regarding function.

The sEMG can also reflect quantitative estimation on the basis of a maximal voluntary contraction (MVC) reference (Disselhorst-Klug et al., 2009). Often the sEMG data is combined with other data (e.g. gait) to gain a better understanding of overall neuromuscular performance. The sEMG has also been used to study fatigue, particularly during repeated trials to examine relative changes due to fatigue (Disselhorst-Klug et al., 2009).

Measurement Techniques

The reliability of EMG measurements is dependent on several factors including the type of electrode used, electrode placement and velocity, magnitude of muscle contraction, nature of signal processing, and frequency response of the recording equipment (Fabio, 1987). Electrode placement is critical as there is evidence that electrode location can influence muscle action potential conduction velocity and the mean power frequency of the sEMG (Hogrel et al., 1998). Several good guidelines have been developed over the years to provide guidance regarding electrode placement (DeLuca, 1997). The Surface ElectroMyography for the Non-Invasive Assessment of Muscles (SENIAM) project resulted in European recommendations for sensors and sensor placement procedures as well as signal processing methods for sEMG (seniam.org). Researchers should use one of the many published guidelines regarding electrode placement (seniam.org, Criswell, 2011), along with an understanding of the underlying physiology and anatomy, to place electrodes over the optimal recording location. Depending on the type of disorder, the choice of electrode size may vary as well. The SENIAM guidelines indicate that the electrode diameter should be lower than 10 mm, and the distance between electrode centres should less or equal to 20 mm (seniam.org).

There are two sources of motion artefact in surface electrodes; mechanical disturbance of the electrode charge layer and movement of the skin under the electrodes (Clancy et al., 2002). Major sources of contamination in the EMG signal include electrode noise, electrode motion artefact, cable motion artefact, power line interference (60 Hz in North America and 50 Hz in Europe), the instrumentation used to amplify and filter the EMG, and contamination from other biosignals (Clancy et al., 2002).

Careful placement of electrodes, accurate recording instrumentation along with the appropriate signal processing techniques (such as filtering and smoothing) significantly reduce the impact of noise.

Considering the quality of the signal is a key factor when recording sEMG data. In order to reduce error when measuring the signal it is important, as previously discussed, that the electrode skin interface be as conductive as possible. The sEMG is essentially the summation of the motor unit action potentials occurring during the contraction measured at a given electrode location (Leham& McGill, 1999). Standard skin preparation techniques and appropriate electrode configuration can be used to minimize error (De Luca, 1997; seniam.org).

Data Analysis Methods

While obtaining sEMG signals is reasonably easy to collect, the analysis of the signals to obtain useful information can be complicated. For clinicians it is important to determine what questions the sEMG is being used to answer. There are several techniques currently used to examine the signal including time domain analysis, frequency domain analysis, and combined time-frequency analyses (wavelet analysis). Depending on the type of information sought and the application of interest, one or more types of analysis may be needed.

Amplitude Estimation

With respect to time domain analysis two methods are consistently used. The first is to use the sEMG to estimate the amplitude of the signal as a representation of the amount of muscle activity generated during a contraction (activation level) and to estimate force. The second method examines the duration of the individual muscle activity to study timing patterns.

The EMG amplitude can be defined as the time-varying standard deviation of the EMG (Clancy et al., 2002). Objective amplitude measurements of the sEMG have been attempted with various physical therapy interventions including splinting, isokinetic dynamometry, exercise, biofeedback and gait (Fabio, 1987). Amplitude estimation can be accomplished through a variety of methods (Basmajian& DeLuca, 1985). Commonly used techniques to estimate amplitude include signal averaging, smoothing, and calculation of an integrated EMG, rectification and calculation of the root mean square value. Averaging the signal involves producing a mean of several trials of performance of the same motor act. The average of 'x' points are then averaged to reduce the variability of the signal by 'x.' Smoothing is the method of averaging enough to eliminate random fluctuations, similar to removing "bumps" from the signal. Integrated EMG (iEMG) is often reported and simply refers to the total amount of muscle activity occurring during any given time interval as represented by the area under the curve during that time interval. The iEMG increases in slope as long as any EMG activity is present and decreases with less activity during isometric, stationary contractions (Basmajian&DeLuca, 1985). The EMG signal can also be rectified, that is the portion of the signal below the 0 point (the negative electrical potential) is made positive and artificially placed above the zero crossing. Finally, the root mean square (RMS) voltage is often used to estimate the EMG amplitude. The RMS measures the electrical power in the signal and provides an instantaneous measure of the power output of the EMG signal. The EMG signal is squared, then summed and averaged and finally the root of the product is derived. Often the sEMG is used to estimate muscle force, thus better amplitude estimation will result in better EMG-force estimation (Clancy et al., 2002).

Due to the random nature of the EMG signal it is important to consider what the amplitude can be compared to. In order to calibrate the signal, often normalization techniques are used. Normalization involves collecting a baseline signal (often a maximal voluntary contraction, or MVC) under static conditions and comparing it to the sEMG from the test contractions. Normalization techniques are varied when examining dynamic contractions and when clinical populations are studied, this will be discussed at greater length later in this chapter.

Rather than examining the sEMG amplitude values, looking at the presence of amplitude variations (which may account for the ability of the muscle to vary its contraction level in response to variation in mechanical demand) may be more appropriate to assess patients with neurological disease (Merlo &Campanini, 2010).

Force Estimates

The advantage of sEMG is that it is one of the few methods that provide insight on muscle activity and therefore muscle force production during functional movements (Staudenmann et al., 2010). While inverse dynamics analysis allows calculation of the net moment produced by muscles surrounding a joint, it does not allow for calculation of force in individual muscles (Staudenmann et al., 2010). As muscles are not easily accessible to directly measure force, sEMG is often used to estimate force. While there has been much research attempting to quantify force on the basis of surface EMG, interpretation of the signal can be misleading and potentially dangerous (DeLuca, 1997). There have been indications that as isometric muscle force increases (for certain muscles), so too does the amplitude of the EMG signal (Basmajian&DeLuca, 1985, DeLuca, 1997, Disselhorst-Klug et al., 2009), however during dynamic movements this relationship is unclear (Disselhorst-Klug et al., 2009). During gait and generally during movement, this relationship fails (Merlo & Campanini, 2010).

Unlike stationary isometric contractions, dynamic activity involves changes in muscle length. In this case, the sEMG –force relationship is affected by numerous factors including the activation pattern of the motor units, the anatomical, mechanical or electrical properties of the muscle, the location of the surface electrodes relative to the muscle and the properties of the contracting filaments within the cells (Disselhorst-Klug et al., 2009). In reproducible, cyclic activities, such as gait or riding a bicycle, the EMG activity can be used to derive an estimate of force input (Disselhorst-Klug et al., 2009). The absolute force still may not be derived from the signal, however a relative value and changes in those values can be estimated.

Muscle Coordination and Temporal Information

In addition to amplitude measures, the phasic activity of the sEMG is often examined using time domain analysis. sEMG recordings have been used extensively in the study of movement patterns by examining the timing patterns of the muscle activity (Yack, 1984).

This method refers to the times at which the signal is activated and then deactivated (or 'on' and 'off' times). This information is helpful to understand the relative activity of muscles throughout a contraction and is particularly useful to understand the relative muscle activity for clinical populations. Timing data can be examined throughout a dynamic activity and combined with other measures (e.g. gait data) can provide useful information regarding muscle coordination.

An area of interest to physical therapists is the measurement of the quality of movement (Fabio, 1987). One method of determining this is the temporal sequence of muscle activation. There are many methods described for examining the temporal parameters of EMG including scoring by trained examiners and computerized methods. The use of trained examiners generally involves physical therapists trained to identify baseline activity visually and then identify the beginning of EMG activity (i.e. a significant departure from baseline). Computerized methods use a baseline reference of the sEMG samples and then a variety of techniques to determine significant variation from the baseline (e.g. two or three standard deviations from the baseline). It has been shown (Fabio, 1987) that while numerous researchers have used variations of the computerized methods, there remain questions regarding an appropriate threshold level. Newer mathematical techniques have been developed to improve the accuracy of these methods, which may reduce error. In addition, it is useful to combine the sEMG timing data with kinematic data to complement the EMG data (Hug, 2011).

An important area of interest to clinicians is to understand how muscles are coordinated to perform common motor tasks (Hug, 2011). Muscle coordination is defined as "a distribution of muscle activation or force among individual muscles to produce a given combination of joint moments" (Prilutskuy, 2000).

While both EMG and force data can be used to study muscle coordination, it is mainly studied from sEMG activity (Hug, 2011). Studies that examine muscle coordination generally report muscle activity profiles, i.e. the sEMG patterns (Hug, 2011). These patterns provide information regarding the timing of the signal, the shape of the activity and allows for amplitude estimation. Newer approaches such as wavelet transformations decompose the EMG signal into time and frequency intensities for an EMG intensity pattern (von Tscharner&Nigg, 2008). Measuring coordination with sEMG is affected by a number of factors including amplitude cancellation, crosstalk, and spatial variability of muscle activity (Hug, 2011).

The evaluation of muscular co-ordination is particularly of interest to clinicians to better understand movement patterns in clinical groups. Many activities require coordination of the muscles on both sides of a joint, also known as muscle coactivation or co-contraction. Co-contraction is associated with stability (Psek&Cafarelli, 1993) and therefore of great interest to clinicians. In order to measure co-contraction it is necessary to record sEMG signals from multiple muscle sites (agonist, antagonist and synergist muscles). Unfortunately, the measurement from multiple sites is negatively affected by the presence of crosstalk. While crosstalk can be reduced, it can never be completely removed. The presence of crosstalk complicates assessment of muscle co-ordination and estimation of muscle force (Disselhorst-Klug et al., 2009). Some research has used the cross-correlation coefficient to quantify the magnitude of crosstalk (Morrenhof&Abbink, 1985), however recent research has suggested that this method is insufficient (Farina et al., 2002a). Knowing the individual crosstalk risk factor allows for more reliable assessment in this case (Disselhorst-Klug et al., 2009). The crosstalk risk factor introduced by Meinecke et al. (2004) allows one to distinguish between crosstalk and muscular coactivation (Disselhorst-Klug et al., 2009).

Research has shown that the sEMG is useful for examining co-contraction in clinical populations. There is evidence that co-contraction magnitude and total EMG magnitude have an inverse relationship to energy expenditure (measured via heart rate monitoring) in children with spastic CP. In addition, it has been shown that children with more muscle activity in the agonist and antagonist tended to be more energy efficient (Damiano et al., 2000). This research was significant as it used the sEMG data to determine the activation strategies used by children affected by CP that directly impact motor function.

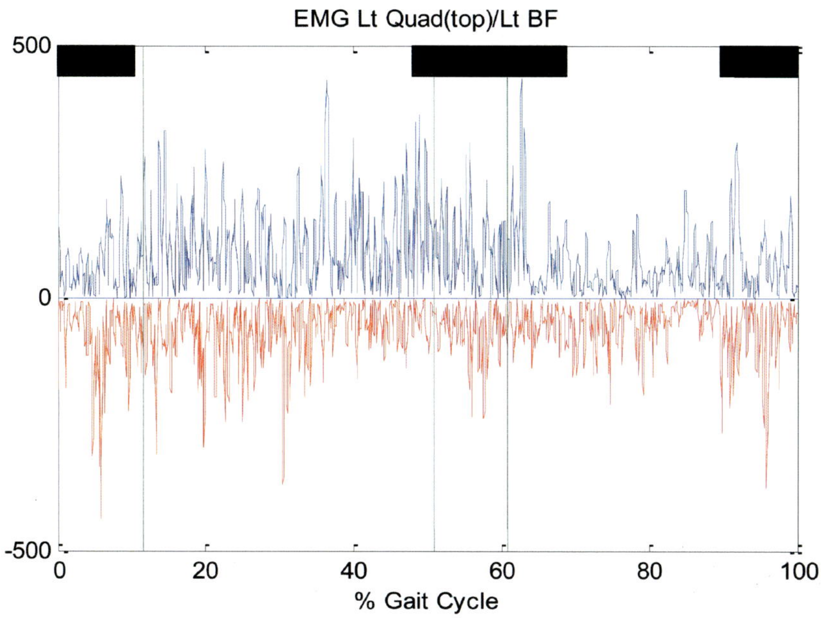

Figure 3. Cocontraction plot of rectus femoris (blue) activity and biceps femoris (red) activity plotted versus percentage of gait cycle. Black bars represent the typical onset and offset times of the rectus femoris muscle. Key gait cycle events are marked with green dashed lines (opposite toe-off, opposite foot strike, toe-off).

Figure 3 illustrates co-contraction graphically. The upper signal represents the muscle activity of the rectus femoris while the lower signal represents the activity of the biceps femoris across a typical gait cycle. As can be seen, the antagonist biceps femoris are clearly activated throughout the gait cycle for this individual. This type of muscle activation pattern is useful for clinicians to determine rehabilitation protocols for patients.

Normalization

When sEMG data is processed in the time domain (e.g. amplitude estimation) and then compared between trials that require reapplication of electrodes, between muscles, or between individuals, they need to be normalized (De Luca, 1997; Burden, 2010). Normalization of the signal is the process of expressing the activity in relation to a calibrated test contraction. Normalization of EMGs is required due to the many technical, anatomical and physiological factors that can influence the magnitude of the signal and due to the inherent instability of the signal (De Luca, 1997). The most often used method of normalization is to compare the test contraction activity against a standardized maximal voluntary contraction (MVC). The difficulty of this method is ensuring that subjects are truly exerting maximal force during the test. This method is further compromised when conducting experiments with clinical subjects as they may not be able to produce a MVC from the muscle of interest. Submaximal contractions have been used as reference levels with limited success (Lehman & McGill, 1999). Furthermore, the use of an isometric MVC as a reference to which dynamic data is compared brings up the question of validity. Some researchers have used maximal values during dynamic activity as the reference data for normalization, again with limited success.

A unanimous normalization procedure has not been identified as of yet (Friggo&Crenna, 2009, Hug, 2011), however different methods have been proposed (Yang and Winter, 1984, Burden et al., 2003). Current normalization methods can only be used to obtain an approximate degree of muscle activity or to determine the major muscles involved in a given movement (Hug, 2011). However, it is generally accepted that normalization is required in spite of its lack of precision (Hug, 2011). There is a need to further examine the issue of normalization, particularly with clinical groups, to determine the most appropriate technique.

Spectral Estimation

Frequency domain analysis (spectral estimation) can also be used to examine the sEMG. The most widely used method for spectral estimation is the Fourier transform and the fast FT (FFT) algorithm (Karlsson et al., 2009). Shifts in frequency parameters such as mean or median frequency have been used as indicators of muscle fatigue (De Luca, 1997, Basmajian& De Luca, 1985, Merletti& Parker, 2004).

Muscle fatigue may be accompanied by changes in muscle electrical activity (Dimitrova&Dimitrova, 2003). Muscle fatigue is a decrease in the maximal force or power that the involved muscles can produce due to one (or several) physiological processes that enable the contractile proteins to generate force becoming impaired (Enoka&Duchateau, 2008). Muscle fatigue is complex and the underlying causes of the fatigue are vast including both central and peripheral causes. Much research has surrounded methods to estimate fatigue under various conditions, however there remain many unanswered questions including determining the exact cause of the fatigue (Dimitrova&Dimitrova, 2003).

While there are several methods that can be used to estimate muscle fatigue, including time domain methods (estimates to the sEMG amplitude, zero-crossing rate of the signal and spike analysis) as well as frequency domain methods such as signal spectrum compression (Ciftrek et al., 2009) the most common method is the use of spectral parameters. The mean frequency of the power spectrum is often used to quantify muscular fatigue (Lindstrom et al., 1977; Merletti et al., 1990) and a shift to lower frequencies has been suggested to be due to a decrease in the action potential conduction velocity (Merletti et al., 1990). An example of this phenomenon is shown in Figure 4. The spectral parameters associated with fatigue have been shown to be influenced by various factors including longitudinal position of the electrodes (Dimitrova&Dimitrova, 2003).

The joint analysis of the EMG spectrum and amplitude parameters has been shown to be a useful method in those situations where fatigue and recovery trade off (e.g. occupational settings). In this analysis it has been suggested that four different cases can be identified: 1) if the EMG amplitude increases and the EMG spectrum shifts to the right, muscle force is likely the cause of the fatigue, 2) if the EMG amplitude decreases and the EMG spectrum shifts to the left, muscle force decrease is the likely cause, 3) if the EMG amplitude increases and EMG spectrum shifts to the left, this is likely the result of muscle fatigue and 4) if the EMG amplitude decreases and the EMG spectrum shifts to the right, this may be recovery from previous muscle fatigue (Ciftrek et al., 2009).

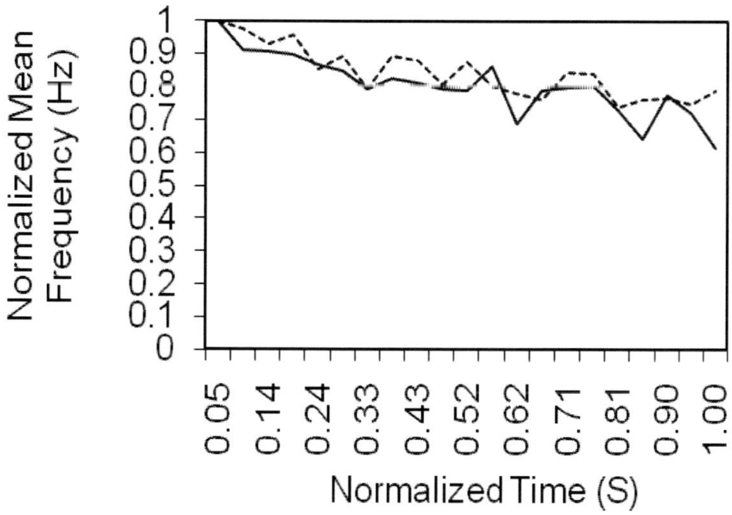

Figure 4. Example of frequency shifts due to fatigue. The data represents fatigue in the quadriceps femoris muscle during an isometric knee extension. The power spectrum was computed. The mean frequency (MF) was then calculated every 2 seconds and the decline in the MF over time is evident.

The basic assumption of the FFT, however is that the signal is stationary. Most contractions in daily life are not static or stationary, therefore for the study of dynamic contractions newer methods such as time-frequency analysis have been used to varying degrees of success.

Time-frequency and Wavelet Analyses

Because the FFT that assumes a stationary signal and therefore is not necessarily valid in dynamic activities, newer methods of analysis have been developed. Time-frequency methods such as quadratic time-frequency representations that do not require stationarity (Ciftrek et al., 2009) have become popular methods of analyses.

Wavelet analysis has been used in many applications in medicine and biology (von Tscharner, 2000). It has been suggested that the sEMG contains more information than what is calculated in root mean square analysis (amplitude estimation) or in the power spectrum. Intensity analysis uses time-frequency analysis to represent a quantitative analysis that approximates the power of the EMG signal at time *t* (von Tscharner, 2000). The advantage of this type of analysis is that it indicates less about the detail of the EMG signal and more about the detail with respect to the functional aspects of muscle activation (von Tscharner, 2000).

The wavelet transformation can be used to decompose the EMG signal into its intensities, both time and frequency. Unlike traditional frequency domain analysis, which due to its assumption of stationarity requires analysis of very short time epochs, the wavelet transformation can be used for frequency analysis of muscle activation during various dynamic exercises (Friggo&Crenna, 2009). The wavelet transformation has been used to assess EMG timing during gait (Merlo et al., 2003), compare gait analysis between children with cerebral palsy and normally developing children (Lauera et al. 2005) and for the classification of EMG patterns (Engelhart et al., 1999).

Integrating Biomechanical Data with sEMG

Biomechanical analyses typically involve kinematic and kinetic analyses of movement. Kinematic data describes motion using temporal-spatial parameters (e.g. movement timing) and linear and angular parameters (e.g. angles, velocities, accelerations). Kinetic data refers to the underlying forces and moments that cause movement. Using an inverse dynamics approach, kinetic data is obtained by combining kinematic data, ground reaction force data, and segment inertia data. Using this technique, one can compute the *net* joint moments and powers at each joint in the mechanical model. However, net activity does not provide information on individual muscle activity. Therefore, EMG plays a critical role in helping researchers and clinicians understand which muscles contributed to the overall net kinetics. In order to understand the control strategies used for any given task, the muscle activity during a task must be studied (Kleissen et al., 1998) and this can be accomplished with sEMG.

Graphical Representation of EMG Signals

It is imperative that if sEMG is employed in a clinical setting, the data is represented in a manner that is easy to use by clinicians. In addition to high-level signal processing techniques (spectral estimation, wavelet transformation), graphical representation of the data is useful. As previously discussed, timing analysis can provide information regarding the on/off patterns of various muscles. These can be represented numerically with onset and offset times (in mS). Figure 5 shows how these data can then be translated to represent visual onset/offset of muscles over a gait cycle. Figure 6 provides another graphical representation of the sEMG over a gait cycle and includes percent activation expected from the muscle.

Combining the graphical data with details of a particular case can also provide significant information to the clinician for their assessment. Figure 7 illustrates the use of sEMG in case studies to be presented to a clinical team for evaluation.

Applications of sEMG in Clinical Populations

The sEMG has been shown to be a useful tool for clinical populations. The sEMG can be used to examine deviations from normal motor unit firing patterns, to identify muscles for transfer, and to evaluate surgical outcomes (Wren et al., 2006). While muscle timing can be quantified using onset and offset times and amplitude can be quantified, often muscle activity during gait is assessed through subjective visual examination by clinicians (Wren et al., 2006). The limitations of the visual method are the subjective nature of the test and that the information about the shape of the EMG signals is ignored across the gait cycle (Wren et al., 2006). It has been shown that cross-correlation may be useful for evaluating changes in an individuals patient's muscle activation patterns (e.g. before and after surgery), but not for comparing EMG patterns among different individuals such as between patients and normative data (Wren et al., 2006).

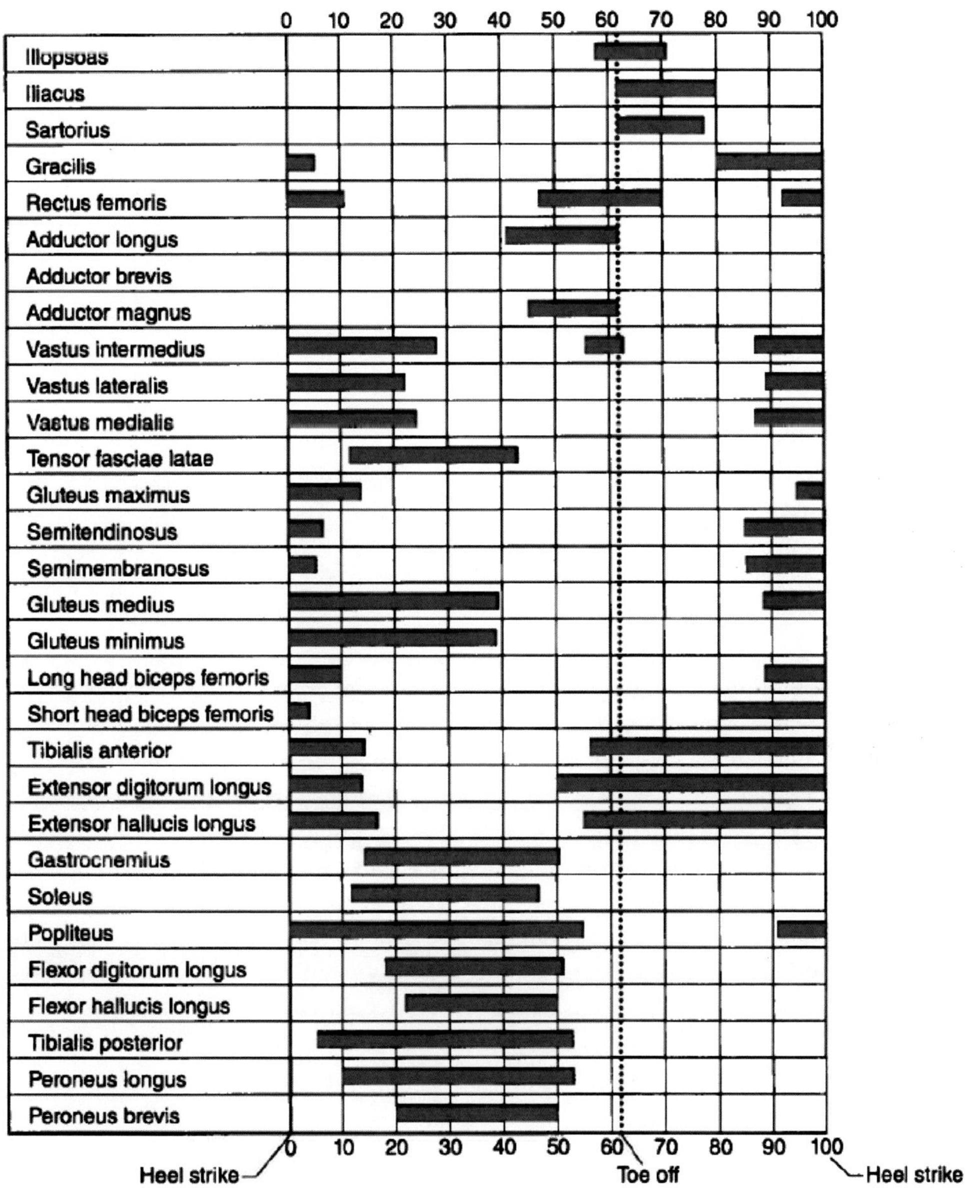

Figure 5. Onset/offset of muscles during gait cycle. (From: Gage, 2004, reprinted with permission).

While sEMG has certain limitations, it can be considered a complementary tool to other movement assessment tools as well as to needle EMG (Hogrel, 2005). sEMG applications in neurology include both central and peripheral nervous system (Zwarts et al., 2000). In the central nervous system, the sEMG can be used to measure timing, movement patterns, amount of activity or central drive, involuntary movements, central fatigue and tremor. In the peripheral nervous system, the sEMG can be used to examine evoked activity and voluntary activity, fatigue, muscle fibre conduction velocity and motor unit potential variables including amplitude and duration (Zwarts et al., 2000). The use of sEMG during gait, and during movement in general, can provide useful information the in the planning of treatment for patients with upper motor neuron syndrome (Merlo &Campanini, 2010). It has also been shown that sEMG can be used to examine differences in postural control and movement performance during goal directed reaching (Johnston, et al., 2002).

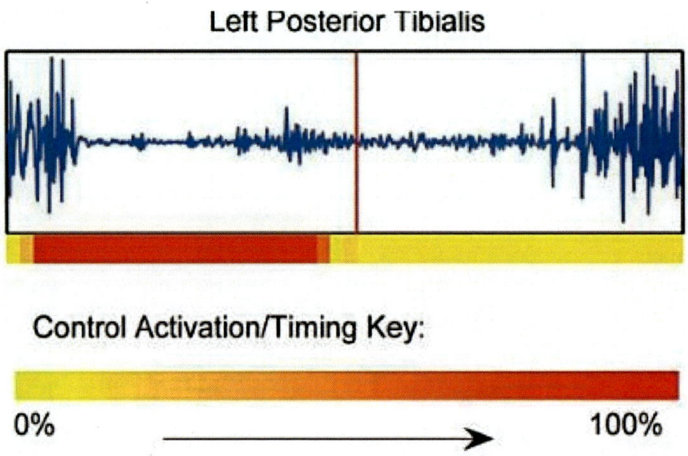

Figure 6. EMG data for the tibialis posterior during a gait cycle. The expected activation of the muscle is depicted by colour bands. For this patient, the muscle is relatively quiet when it should be active and vice versa. (From: Gage, 2009, reprinted with permission).

Clinics are increasingly using sEMG recordings of movement data to aid in pre-surgical planning and in outcome assessment (Perry et al., 2001). Often the data is assessed by the temporal (on/off) behaviour of muscles. There has been a push to integrate motion data with sEMG and this type of integrated data can lead to more extensive analysis of the movement (Perry et al., 2001). In addition, while gait research concentrates on ambulatory movement (i.e. walking), sEMG and motion analysis have great benefit to understanding motor tasks performed by clinical patients in non-ambulatory conditions. There have been promising results suggesting that the sEMG can be used for quantifying muscle activity during voluntary motor tasks in non-ambulatory children with CP (Perry et al., 2001).

Research has shown that in some instances the sEMG is more accurate than needle EMG for the detection of spontaneous activity in subjects with several neuropathies (Hogrel, 2005). This was attributed to the ability to record the sEMG for an increased length of time that is not possible with needle electrodes. Studies that have compared surface and fine wire EMG signals have found greater reliability with surface electrodes (Young, Rose, & Biden, 1989; Giroux &Lamontagne, 1990; Kadaba et al., 1985). This is likely a function of the small volume of tissue that is tested.

Spectral parameters of the sEMG, such as median frequency, have been used to examine muscle fatigue during sustained isometric contractions, however the relationship with fatigue is much more complicated during anisometric contractions (Hogrel, 2005, De Luca, 1997, Merletti& Parker, 2004). Another parameter of sEMG of use to clinicians is the analysis of propagation, or the estimation of muscle fibre conduction velocity. In this type of analysis, the signal between at least two sites (having the same alignment as the muscle fibres) is measured. It has been shown that the MFCV may be reduced in clinical populations such as those suffering from Duchenne muscular dystrophy, myotonicdystrophy, McArdle's disease or congenital myopathy (Hogrel, 2005). In patients with ALS, it has been shown that the MFCV is significantly increased compared with controls (Zwarts et al., 2000).

In clinical gait analysis, sEMG data is collected simultaneously with kinematic and kinetic descriptors of locomotor movements (Frigo&Crenna, 2009). EMG devices that use cables or wires to tether the subject to the data collection system could interfere with natural movement patterns. Similarly, for pediatric researchers, the weight of data packs placed on patients may cause movement changes. The advent of wireless sEMG systems has improved the methods of data collection by eliminating these cumbersome wires and allowing unrestrained movement. For example, the 16-bit Zerowire system by Aurion (Figure 8) uses lightweight, signal processing and power transmission units. Data is transmitted through the WiFi band to the receiver, which is connected directly to a PC.

Natural movement patterns and wireless EMG equipment may also be needed for other gross motor activities such as sit-to-stand, gymnastics, running, and workplace simulations. Fine motor activities and research involving object manipulation may also benefit from wireless systems.

Clinical Case Study:

Amy is an 11-year-old female patient with spastic diplegic cerebral palsy. She is diagnosed with stiff knee (tight and spastic rectus femoris) and crouch (very tight and spastic hamstrings). Amy frequently falls due to problems clearing the limb during the swing phase of gait. Stiff-knee patterns are likely due to excessive knee joint moments in double support and low knee flexion velocity at toe-off (Goldberg et al., 2006). An overactive rectus femoris may contribute to this excessive moment and must be validated by EMG. In Amy's case, the EMG showed abnormal activity and she later underwent a rectus femoris transfer (Perry, 1987; Gage et al., 1987) to reduce the excessive moment. Post-operatively, range of motion at the knee improved during both the stance and swing phase of gait.

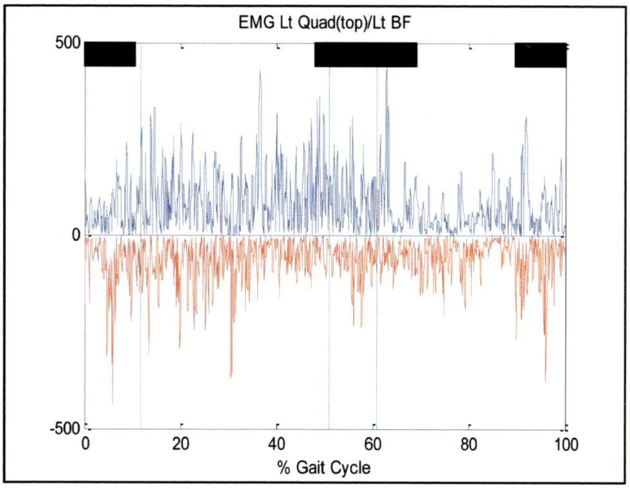

Figure 7. Clinical Case Study: Agonist/antagonist plot of the rectus femoris and semimembranosus activity during a gait cycle. Black bars at the top of the figure show the normative timing and duration of rectus femoris activity. Amy demonstrated continuous activity of the rectus femoris throughout the gait cycle.

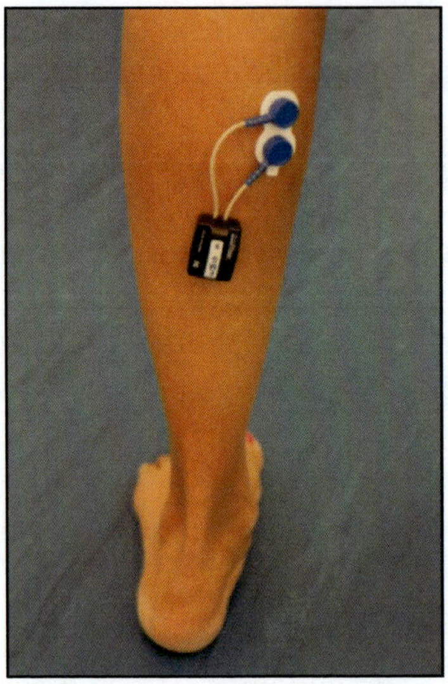

Figure 8. Example of wireless EMG system. There are many wireless surface EMG systems now available on the market. This figure illustrates the ease of using these systems to capture EMG from clinical patients.

EMG Challenges with Clinical Groups

Data Interpretation

While sEMG has been used successfully in the clinical setting, there are a number of challenges. A review by Hogrel (2005) discusses many of the current limitations of clinically based sEMG measures. The potential benefits of using this non-invasive technique for clinical applications depend on the quality of the measurement (Hogrel, 2005). The difficulty of using sEMG is reliability and interpretation of the data. There are a number of variables that can influence the signal and it is imperative that these are considered and addressed in order to limit error. In order to avoid biasing data it has been suggested that the modifying factors can be classified according to their level of influence on the signal as; technical level, experimental level, descriptive level and physiological level (Hogrel, 2005). The technical level is described as environmental conditions and technical specifications of the recording equipment. The experimental level refers to the measurement procedures such as skin preparation and electrode configuration. The descriptive level encompasses the signal processing used, while the physiological level refers to the physiological characteristics of the neuromuscular system. In spite of these concerns, the sEMG can be a useful tool for clinicians to integrate into routine use.

Researchers often use the detected sEMG signal to estimate global muscle activity, however misinterpretation is possible, and in many cases likely. While various parameters can be extracted from the signal (e.g. signal amplitude, power spectrum and onset of muscular activities), it is often unclear what underlying effects they depend on (Rau et al., 2004). For example, the on- and off-times of muscles are often used in clinical applications to examine muscular co-ordination patterns of different muscles. However, the method to use to detect the onset of muscular activity correctly is still being discussed (Rau et al., 2004). In addition, crosstalk between different muscles can impact the timing information. The development of "expert-assist systems" can overcome some of these limitations. These expert systems use a fuzzy-interference methodology to make predictions that support the interpretation of muscular co-ordination patterns and reduce the number of variables to make the sEMG information more accessible for clinicians (Rau et al., 2004). There is promise for this type of approach to extracting meaningful data from the sEMG.

Pathology

One of the difficulties of using sEMG with clinical patient is the complexity of their pathology. The ability to obtain quality signals is complicated if the underlying musculature has been injured or, in the case of amputees, missing. If a patient has more than one disease or disorder, their pathology becomes more complex. Factors such as age and injury also can complicate a patient's pathology. It is important that clinicians examine a patient's pathology to determine if sEMG can a) be reliably collected and b) provide insight above other types of clinical tests. A simple model to describe the role of movement analysis in the clinical process was proposed by Kleissen et al. (1998). In this model a patient with a health problem comes to the clinical institute for treatment. Then, when treatment is completed and the health problem is solved, the patient leaves the institute. It is up to the clinician to select the most suitable treatment for the patient depending on the patient's pathology. In order to this, a reliable patient assessment is needed. Movement analysis techniques, including sEMG observation, could be part of this assessment process. Once the assessment is complete, treatment is recommended and provided, during which time progress is monitored. Movement analysis data can provide objective and quantitative data during this process as well (Kleissen et al., 1998).

Signal Quality and Reliability

Another challenge with obtaining sEMG from clinical groups is recording high quality signals. Due to the nature of collecting the signal from the muscle surface, the quality of the signal is highly dependent on the muscle structure and underlying tissues. It is difficult to obtain good quality signals from those muscles that are small or deep within tissue. Signal quality can also be compromised due previous injury, disease, or disorder. For example, depending on the type of amputation suffered by an individual, the residual muscle may or may not be sufficient to obtain consistent sEMG for use with a powered prosthesis. Similarly, if a patient has suffered many surgeries, the location of muscle and surrounding scar tissue can make it difficult to obtain good signals. Crosstalk between muscles that can contaminate the recorded signal is a concern for both healthy and clinical populations however depending on the type of disorder may be inevitable further compromising the signal. In spite of these concerns, much research has used sEMG with clinical populations to gain a greater insight into muscle function. Provided the researcher understands the limitations of sEMG and considers how the signal is recorded, sEMG can provide valuable information to clinicians.

Electrode placement is also critical for reliable data collection. Placement is dependent on locating muscles accurately and often obtaining good quality data from clinical subjects can be challenging. Changes in muscle architecture due to disease, disorder or injury can impact the placement of electrodes and the quality of the recorded signal. While many guidelines exist for electrode placement (seniam.org, Criswell, 2011), these suggestions were developed using healthy muscle. Clinicians and researchers must take care when applying these placement guidelines to individuals who may have compromised muscle architecture. For example, when collecting data from amputees depending on the length of the residual limb, the site from which sEMG is recorded could be limited. The quality of the sEMG is also dependent on the underlying tissue. If the muscle of interest is hampered by significant subcutaneous tissue, the quality of the signal recorded will be diminished. In addition, if an individual requires an assistive device (e.g. leg brace) and sEMG is to be studied during gait, it may be difficult to place surface electrodes so as to not interfere with the device. The advent of wireless systems has greatly increased the types of research studied by removing cumbersome wires that can interfere with completion of tasks. The use of these systems along with creativity in placement of electrodes is often needed to obtain good signals from clinical patients. Newer multi-channel high density EMG systems, with up to 123 channels of monopolar electrodes, have also reduced the need for exact placement of electrodes and increased the amount of information that can be extracted (Frigo&Crenna, 2009). These systems provide temporal and spatial information that can be used to create maps of limbs that do not depend on electrodes being placed precisely over the muscle of interest. The research in this field has been promising, but the use of these systems with clinical groups has, to date, been very limited.

In addition to muscle location, one of the concerns of recording meaningful sEMG from clinical patients is the reliability of the measure itself. Electrode placement is critical for accurate measurement and this placement is hampered by any assistive technology that may interfere (e.g. patients that use braces to aid in walking). In addition, it is simply not practical to use a system with cumbersome wires that may affect their completion of movements. Developments in wireless technology have alleviated some of these concerns (Figure 8). Impact of previous injury, disease disorder (effects on electrode placement, etc.).

Repeatability

While it has become easier to obtain signals from a muscle, there are challenges obtaining detailed, repeatable, reliable and meaningful results (Rau et al., 2004) which is a concern with clinical groups. Repeatability of sEMG signals can be different according to the category of subject being studied (Friggo and Crenna, 2009).

Granata et al. (2005) have shown that within-session variability of sEMG waveforms in children is much higher than that observed in adults, while between session variability was very similar in the two age groups.

It is imperative that when studying clinical groups the method of data collection and processing is standardized. Kleissen et al. (1997) showed that subjects that were examined in three different gait laboratories showed very similar EMG results including the times of peak, onset and cessation of EMG activity were repeatable within few percent of the gait cycle.

One of the disadvantages of sEMG is that conventional surface electrodes have limited spatial resolution and detect a superposition of a very large number of motor units (Rau et al., 2004). High spatial resolution sEMG using one- or two-dimensional electrode arrays have shown promise in this aspect, as have newer, multichannel high-density EMG systems.

Fatigue

A concern with interpreting sEMG data is the inherent instability and variability of the signal. One concern is the impact of neuromuscular fatigue, which can affect the interpretation of the EMG data (Hug, 2011).

Clinical populations may have difficulty completing the movements to be studied, and may suffer fatigue throughout the movement making any interpretation of the recorded EMG difficult. This is particularly challenging when studying pediatric groups.

Analysis Methods

Clinicians tend to use three main characteristics of the sEMG signal: timing, morphology and amplitude assessment (Merlo &Campanini, 2010). For clinical groups, different physiological and neuromuscular challenges are present. When studying gait cycles, errors in the identification of key events such as the beginning and end of the cycle, walking speed, pain, limb rotation with respect to the direction of the movement, muscle overactivity, altered recruitment, and muscle shortening may be affected by subject-specific factors (Merlo &Campanini, 2010).

Depending on the factor, the impact on the sEMG data differs. For example, variations in walking speed primarily affect the sEMG amplitude more so than phasic (timing) data (Den Otter et al., 2004). Pain can alter muscle patterns if patient alters movement to avoid the pain (Merlo &Campanini, 2010). Limb rotation may alter the functional effect of muscles and lever arms and therefore muscle onset may change according to the biomechanical configuration (Merlo &Campanini, 2010).

There is promising data published using advanced signal processing techniques such as wavelet analysis with clinical populations, particularly children. Wavelet analyses provide a more comprehensive evaluation of sEMG data with the limitations of the FFT, which requires a stationary signal.

Lauera (2005) processed EMG data collected during gait trials using the continuous wavelet transform to determine if a quantitative assessment scale of motor function could be created from the time-frequency information collected. Principle Component Analysis (PCA) was then used to analyze the differences between the instantaneous mean frequency of each group and showed significant deviations in the muscular activity of the child with CP. That study was limited due to the size of the sample population. Wavelet analysis has also been used to distinguish the behaviour of EMG data during the ballistic movements of individuals with Parkinson's disease (Michele, 2003).

Limitations in Literature

EMG Challenges in Pediatric Groups

Surface EMG provides a simple, non-invasive method to estimate muscular activity in children. However, as with any testing procedure, children often pose a challenge for placement of instrumentation and compliance with testing protocols. Accurate placement of EMG electrodes may be difficult due to movement of the child during preparation. Younger children may also alter or remove equipment during testing. Covering the top surface of the electrode with tape and adhering it to the skin may prevent this. In addition, the small size of pediatric limbs contributes to the challenge of accurate electrode placement.

a) Surface vs. Fine Wire Electrodes in Pediatrics

There has been controversy over the use of surface electrodes for measuring muscle activity in children. While fine wire electrodes facilitate localized muscle recordings and reduce crosstalk, this technique is also associated with longer subject preparation times, pain, discomfort, and increased tone in persons with spasticity (Ounpuu et al., 1997). For studies measuring motion (e.g. gait analysis) in addition to EMG, it is possible that pain and discomfort could affect movement patterns. As with adults, the major concern with fine wire EMG is crosstalk or motor unit activity stemming from adjacent or deeper muscles to the muscle of interest. However, this is especially concerning in pediatric populations with small muscle and limb sizes. Ounpuu et al. (1997) examined whether surface EMG could adequately measure muscle activity in the rectus femoris, vastuslateralis, and vastusmedialis in children during muscle isolation tests and gait. Results showed that surface EMG is an appropriate technique for measuring rectus femoris activity if using less than or equal to 2.5cm interelectrode distances. In the case of vastusmedialis and lateralis, less than 0.5cm interelectrode distances were recommended. Similarly, Byrne et al. (2005) studied cross-talk between the rectus femoris and vastuslateralis in five adults. Surface and fine wire EMG were collected simultaneously while subjects performed static contractions consisting of knee extensions and hip flexions. During knee extensions, increased rectus femoris surface activity was found in the absence of fine wire activity. Byrne et al. concluded that this muscular activity most likely originated from the vastusintermedius. The utility of surface EMG and the issue of cross-talk has long been debated (Kadaba et al., 1985; Solomonow et al., 1994) and continues to be a prevalent topic of discussion.

b) EMG Reliability in Pediatrics

Reliability of the sEMG is critical when examining clinical groups. The type of movement being examined will affect the level of repeatability.Granata, Padua, and Abel (2005) examined the repeatability of surface EMG in children during gait. Using the variance ratio, they found that between-day variability for the pediatric group was similar to previously published adult data (Kadaba et al., 1985). However, the pediatric group demonstrated a similar level of variability within-day, which was twice the variability of the adult group. Such variability should be considered when evaluating EMG data within and across testing sessions.

Oksanen et al. (2007) examined intratester reliability of the EMG signals obtained from the neck muscles of adolescents during maximal isometric force contractions. Using intraclass correlation and coefficient of variation measures, intratester reliability was found to be acceptable. The results of this work were consistent with adult studies of neck musculature (Ylinen et al., 1999, 2004; Valkeinen et al., 2002).

Normalization

While normalization of the sEMG data to some calibrated value is recommended (DeLuca, 1997; seniam.org), this procedure can be difficult with children and clinical populations, and in some cases actually introduce error (Feltham, 2010). The choice of calibration level (MVC vs. submaximal contractions, isometric vs. dynamic conditions) complicates the issue. Generally the current normalization procedures are only appropriate for healthy and trained adults (Smith et al., 2008; Van Dieen et al., 2003). If a MVC is chosen for normalization, it has been shown to cause different motor behaviour in children with spastic hemiparetic cerebral palsy (SHCP) compared to a functional task (Van DerWeel et al., 1995; Ricken et al., 2005). Traditional normalization techniques can introduce systematic error because of an inability to perform maximal contractions and therefore invalidates the procedure (Feltham et al., 2010; Van Dieen et al., 2003). Research has shown that the neuromuscular activation of children with SHCP and typically developing children can be assessed on the basis of the mean EMG intensity after it has been smoothed (Feltham et al., 2010). It was found that while this procedure does include some random error and can affect the statistical power due to relatively large between subject variability, it does not threaten the validity of the measurement (Feltham et al., 2010).

In adult studies, EMG data is often normalized by measuring maximum voluntary contractions (MVC) for each muscle of interest. In children, it may be difficult to obtain reliable estimates of the MVC. In addition, such tests may not be feasible for clinical populations with abnormal muscle tone or bony deformities (e.g. cerebral palsy). There is no standard normalization procedure at the present time for clinical populations when making sEMG comparisons.

Traditional EMG vs. Multichannel EMG

Traditionally, sEMG is collected using a bipolar electrode arrangement. Two nearby electrodes are placed over the muscle of interest and a differential amplifier is used to minimize noise. One of the limitations of traditional sEMG is that the resulting signal reflects the activity of the muscles directly below the detecting electrodes. Different types of EMG systems have been developed over the years to improve upon the amount of data that is collected. A linear array of electrodes is a system that detects sEMG signals in a number of points located along a line (Merletti et al., 2003). A spatial filter is usually applied to each point and the resulting data provides information regarding the distribution of the electric potential generated by the activity of the muscle fibers (Merletti et al., 2003). These types of systems have lead to the different applications of the sEMG including identifying anatomical and/or geometrical properties of the motor units, estimation of muscle fiber conduction velocity, sEMG decomposition into classification of single MUAPs, and a better understanding of how signal properties change with increasing distance from the source (Merletti et al., 2003). In clinical applications linear arrays show promise to investigating the conduction properties of motor units (Merletti et al., 2003). Linear arrays involve connecting several bipolar recording electrodes placed in a line, while multichannel sEMG systems increase the number of electrodes and recording positions (Zwarts&Stegeman, 2003). Multichannel EMG systems use high-density EMG grids collect many monopolar EMG signals over a relatively small collection surface (Staudenmann, et al., 2006; Drost et al., 2006). The signals can be examined in different ways, one common method is post-hoc construction of electrode configurations, such as bipolar (Staudenmann, et al., 2006). The monopolar signals can also be considered a multidimensional dataset that likely contains redundant information. Statistical methods such as principal component analysis (PCA) can then be used to detect these redundancies.

Using multiple electrodes with small inter-electrode distances over a muscle, spatiotemporal profiles of individual motor unit potentials (MUPs) can be obtained that reflect MU morphology in greater detail than the MUP shape obtained from a single electrode (van Dijk et al., 2008). Multichannel sEMG allows for the measurement of topographical information concerning the distribution of the EMG activity over a muscle or the timing relationships between different muscles (Zwarts&Stegeman, 2003).

Both multichannel sEMG and linear array electrodes may provide better insight into the mechanisms of the neuromuscular system. The use of these multiple, spatially distributed EMG channels, collecting independent information from separate sources should improve the estimation of muscle force (Staudenmann et al., 2006). This is an important issue in biomechanics and kinesiology as muscle forces cannot be calculated directly and can only be measured using invasive procedures (Staudenmann et al., 2010). While multichannel EMG systems can be used to predict the force output of a muscle, the result appears to be dependent on the method in which the EMG signal is recorded as well as how the signal is processed post-hoc (Staudenmann et al., 2006).

The advantage of high-density multichannel EMG systems is the availability of upwards of 30 channels for data collection (Figure 9).

HD sEMG have been used to better predict muscle activation and estimated force compared to other EMG systems (Staudenmann et al., 2005) and to complement temporal information of the sEMG signal with spatial information (Blok et al., 2005). The information collected from HD sEMG systems can be used to create topographical maps of EMG amplitude at each electrode location and to examine the muscle activity patterns during different tasks (Merletti& Parker, 2004). Recently topographical maps from HD sEMG data were used to research myoelectric control, however that study did not include amputee subjects (Nagata et al., 2007). Recently it was shown that amputee subjects are able to elicit distinct and repeatable patterns for at least a subset of the movements suggesting promise for amputee control of multifunction myoelectric prosthetics (Daley et al., 2010).

In spite of the promising results with clinical groups, there is limited research using HD sEMG with these populations. The ability to record spatial data and gain better insight of the underlying musculature warrants more clinical research with these systems.

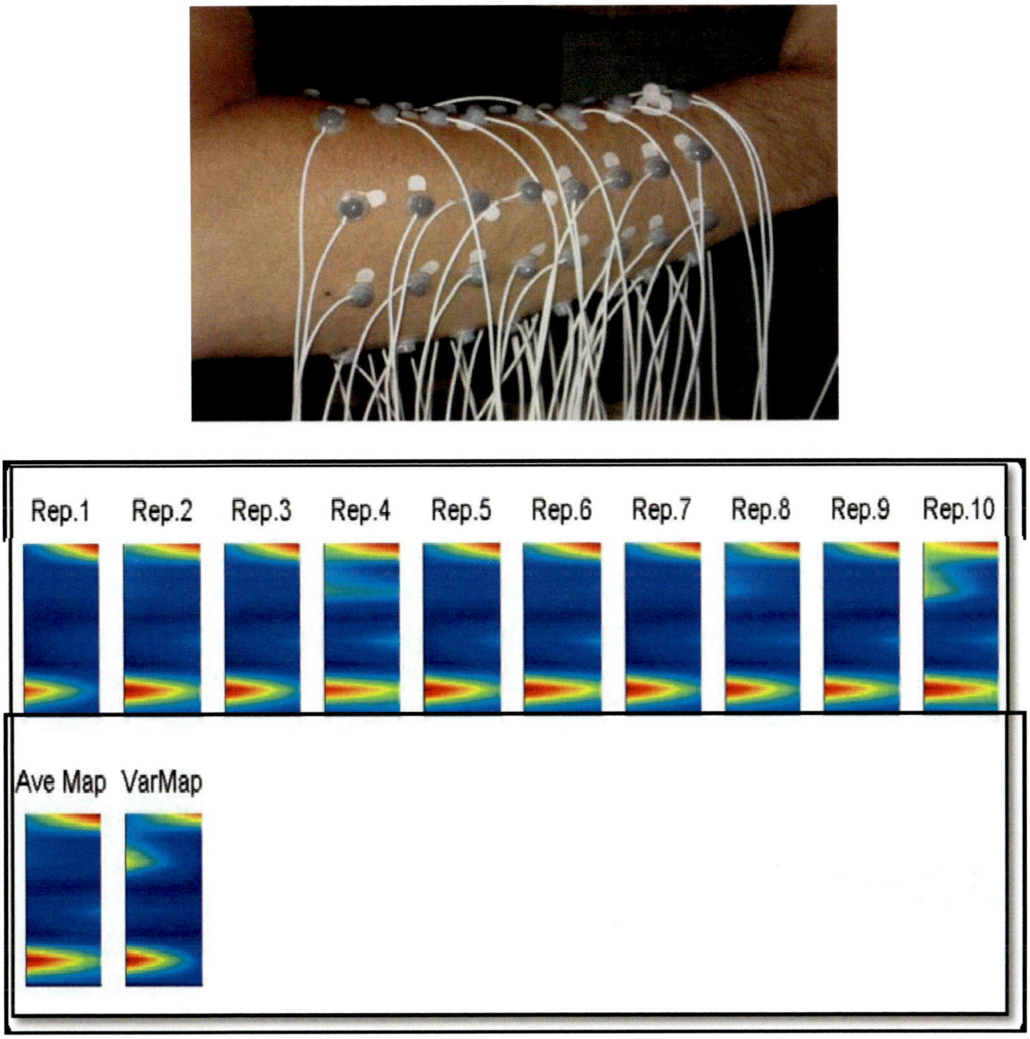

Figure 9. HD EMG System and Corresponding Energy Map. Muscle activity patterns across the 20 repetitions of an upper limb contraction for a congenital amputee. Data showed similar patterns to those produced by normally limbed subjects, with greater variability in energy concentrations.

Conclusion

Surface EMG is a powerful tool for examining muscle activity and movement patterns in healthy and clinical individuals. There have been numerous advances improving the instrumentation used including wireless systems and powerful multichannel recording units. However, care must be taken when incorporating sEMG into clinical assessments. The reliability of the measure is directly related to the quality of the recording. Using the technology with clinical groups can impact the accuracy of the data. In addition, while it is relatively easy to record sEMG data, misinterpretation of the data is possible and, without proper understanding of limitations of the signal, likely. A number of precautions can be taken to ensure accurate, high quality signal recordings including proper skin preparation, proper electrode placement and sensitive recording instrumentation. When recording sEMG data from clinical groups it is important to not alter movement patterns due to cumbersome recording equipment. The development of wireless sEMG systems has reduced the movement artefact due to wires, etc. that contaminates the signal and improve the collection of both biomechanical and EMG data.

The development of multichannel EMG systems has greatly changed how signals are detected and processed. These systems reduce the need for exact placement of electrodes, increase the amount of muscular information detected and provide significant temporal and spatial information. While these systems have shown promise, there is a need to increase their use with clinical groups.

While there are limitations and challenges to recording and interpreting sEMG data, there are many benefits to clinical populations. Surface EMG can provide significant data regarding movement patterns that can be used by clinicians to develop better treatment and rehabilitation protocols. The integration of biomechanical data with the sEMG provides clinicians with a more complete view of any movement limitations. The advantage of using sEMG is that it is non-invasive and, used properly, can provide detailed information regarding muscle activity. As movement is impaired due to disease or injury, understanding muscle activity is critical to begin improvement. Surface EMG is a useful tool and can be an integral part of movement analysis for clinical groups.

References

Basmajian, J. & De Luca, C. J. *Muscles Alive*. 5th ed. Baltimore, MD: Williams & Wilkins; 1985.

Blok, J; van Dijk, J; Zwarts, M; Stegeman, D. Motor unit action potential topography and its use in motor unit estimation. *Muscle and Nerve* 200532, 280-291.

Burden, A. How should we normalize electromyograms obtained from healthy participants? What we have learned from over 25 years of research. *Journal of Electromyography and Kinesiology*, 2010 20, 1023-1035.

Byrne, CA; Lyons, GM; Donnelly AE; O'Keeffe DT; Hermens H; Nene A. Rectus femoris surface myoelectric signal cross-talk during static contractions. *Journal of Electromyography and Kinesiology*, 2005 15, 564-575.

Criswell, E. *Cram's Introduction to Surface Electromyography*. 2nd ed. Sudbury, MA: Jones and Bartlett; 2011.

Cifrek, M; Medved, V; Tonkovic, S; Ostojic, S. Surface EMG based muscle fatigue evaluation in biomechanics. *Clinical Biomechanics*, 2009 24, 327-340.

Clancy, E; Morin, E; Merletti, R. Sampling, noise-reduction and amplitude estimation issues in surface electromyography. *Journal of Electromyography and Kinesiology*, 2002 12, 1-16.

Daley, H; Englheart, K; Kuruganti, U. Muscle activation patterns of the forearm: high density electromyography data of normally limbed and transradial amputee subjects. *Journal of Prosthetics & Orthotics*, 2010 22, 244-251.

Damiano, D; Martellotta, T; Sullivan, D; Granata, K; Abel, M. Muscle force production and functional performance in spastic cerebral palsy: relationship of cocontraction. *Archives of Physical Medicine & Rehabilitation*, 2000 81, 895-900.

Den Otter, A; Geurts, A; Mulder, T; Duysens, J. Speed related changes in muscle activity from normal to very slow walking speeds. *Gait and Posture*, 2004 19, 270-278.

De Luca, CJ. The use of surface electromyography in biomechanics. *Journal of Applied Biomechanics*, 1997 13, 135-163.

Dimitrova, N; Dimitrova, G. Interpretation of EMG changes with fatigue: facts, pitfalls, and fallacies. *Journal of Electromyography and Kinesiology*, 2003 13, 13-36.

Disselhorst-Klug, C; Schmitz-Rode, T; Rau, G. Surface electromyography and muscle force: Limits in sEMG-force relationship and new approaches for applications. *Clinical Biomechanics*, 2009 24, 225-235.

Drost, G; Stegeman, DF; van Engelen, BGM; Zwarts, MJ. Clinical application of high-density surface EMG: A systematic review. *Journal of Electromyography and Kinesiology*, 2006 16, 586-602.

Englehart, K; Hudgins, B; Parker, P; Stevenson, M. Classification of the myoelectric signal using time-frequency based representations. *Medical Engineering and Physics*, 1999 21, 431-438.

Enoka, R. *Neuromechanics of Human Movement*. 4th ed. Champaign, IL: Human Kinetics; 2008.

Enoka, R; Duchateau J. Muscle fatigue: what, why and how it influences muscle function. *Journal of Physiology*, 2008 586 (1), 11-23.

Fabio, R. Reliability of computerized surface electromyography for determining the onset of muscle activity. *Physical Therapy*, 1987 67, 43-48.

Farina, D; Merletti, R; Indino, B; Nazzaro, M; Pozzo, M. Surface EMG crosstalk between knee extensor muscles: experimental and model results. *Muscle and Nerve*, 2002a 26, 681-95.

Farina, D; Holobar, A; Merletti, R; Enoka, R. Decoding the neural drive to muscles from the surface electromyogram. *Clinical Neurophysiology*, 2010 121, 1616-1623.

Farina, D; Cescon, C; Merletti, R. Influence of anatomical, physical, and detection system parameters on surface EMG. *BiolCybern*, 2002b 86, 445-56.

Feltham, M; Ledebt, A; Deconinck, F; Savelsbergh, G. Assessment of neuromuscular activation of the upper limbs in children with spastic hemiparetic cerebral palsy during a dynamical task. *Journal of Electromyography and Kinesiology*, 2010 20, 448-456.

Frigo, C; Crenna, P. Multichannel SEMG in clinical gait analysis: A review and state-of-the-art. *Clinical Biomechanics*, 2009 24, 236-245.

Gage, JR; Perry, J; Hicks, RR; Koop, S; Werntz, JR. Rectus femoris transfer to improve knee function of children with cerebral palsy. *Developmental Medicine and Child Neurology*, 1987 29, 159–166.

Gage, JR. *The Treatment of Gait Problems in Cerebral Palsy*. UK: Cambridge University Press; 2004.

Gage, JR; Schwartz MH; Koop SE; Novacheck TF. *The Identification and Treatment of Gait Problems in Cerebral Palsy*. 2nd edition. London, UK: Mac Keith Press; 2009.

Giroux, B; Lamontagne, M. Comparisons between surface electrodes and intramuscular wire electrodes in isometric and dynamic conditions. *Electromyography and Clinical Neurophysiology*, 1990 30(7), 397-405.

Goldberg, SR; Ounpuu, S; Arnold, AS; Gage, JR; Delp, SR. Kinematic and kinetic factors that correlate with improved knee flexion following treatment for stiff-knee gait. *Journal of Biomechanics*, 2006 39, 689-698.

Granata, K; Padua, D; Abel, M. Repeatability of surface EMG during gait in children. *Gait and Posture*, 2005 22, 346-350.

Hodgkin, AL; Huxley, AF. A quantitative description of membrane current and its application to conduction and excitation in nerve. *Journal of Physiology*, 1952 117, 500-544.

Hogrel, J. Clinical applications of surface electromyography in neuromuscular disorders. *Clinical Neurophysiology*, 2005 35, 59-71.

Hug, F. Can muscle coordination be precisely studied by surface electromyography? *Journal of Electromyography and Kinesiology*, 2011 21, 1-12.

Huxley, AF. Muscle structure and theories of contraction. *Progress in Biophysics and Molecular Biology*, 1957 7, 255-318.

Huxley, AF. Mechanics and models of the myosin motor. *Philosophical Transactions of the Royal Society*, 2000 B355, 433-440.

Johnston, LM; Burns, YR; Brauer, SG; Richardson, CA. Differences in postural control and movement performance during goal directed reaching in children with developmental coordination disorder. *Human Movement Science*, 2002 21, 583-601.

Kadaba, MP; Wootten, ME; Gainey, J; Cochran, GVB. Repeatability of phasic muscle activity: Performance of surface and intramuscular wire electrodes in gait analysis. *Journal of Orthopaedic Research*, 1985 3(3), 350-359.

Karlsson, J; Roeleveld, K; Grönlund, C; Holtermann, A; Östlund, N. Signal processing of the surface electromyography to gain insight into neuromuscular physiology. *Philosophical Transactions of the Royal Society A: Mathematical, Physical & Engineering Sciences*, 2009 367, 337-356.

Kleissen, R; Litjens, M; Baten, C; Harlaar, J; Hof, A; Zilvold, G. Consistency of surface EMG patterns obtained during gait from three laboratories using standardized measurement technique. *Gait & Posture*, 1997 6, 200-209.

Kleissen, R; Buurke, J; Harlaar, J; Zilvold, G. Electromyography in the biomechanical analysis of human movement and its clinical application. *Gait and Posture*, 1998 8, 143-158.

Lauera, R; Stackhouse, C; Shewokis, P; Smith, B; Orlina, M; McCarthy, J. Assessment of wavelet analysis of gait in children with typical development and cerebral palsy. *Journal of Biomechanics*, 2005 38, 1351-1357.

Lehman, G; McGill, S. The importance of normalization in the interpretation of surface electromyography: A proof of principle. *Journal of Manipulative and Physiological Therapeutics*, 1999 22, 444-446.

Lehman, G. Clinical considerations in the use of surface electromyography: Three experimental studies. *Journal of Manipulative and Physiological Therapeutics*, 2002 25, 293-299.

Lindström, L; Kadefors, R; Petersén, I. An electromyography index for localized muscle fatigue. *Journal of Applied Physiology*, 1977 43, 750-4.

Meinecke, L; Disselhorst-Klug, C; Rau, G. Crosstalk and co-activation in bipolar surface EMG data: a new methodology for detection, discrimination and quantification. *Gait and Posture*, 2004 20S, S74-S75.

Merletti, R; Parker, PA. *Electromyography: Physiology, Engineering and Noninvasive Applications*. 1st Edition. Hoboken, NJ: John Wiley & Sons, Inc.; 2004.

Merletti, R; Knaflitz, M; De Luca, C. Myoelectric manifestations of fatigue in voluntary and electrically elicited contractions. *Journal of Applied Physiology*, 1990 69, 1810-20.

Merletti, R; Farina, D; Gazzoni, M. The linear electrode array: a useful tool with many applications. *Journal of Electromyography and Kinesiology*, 2002 13, 37-47.

Merlo, A; Farina, D; Merletti, R. A fast and reliable technique for muscle activity detection from surface EMG signals. *IEEE Transactions on Biomedical Engineering*, 2003 50, 316-323.

Merlo, A; Campanini, I. Technical aspects of surface electromyography for clinicians.*The Open Rehabilitation Journal*, 2010 3, 98-109.

Michele, GD; Sello, S; Carboncini, MC; Rossi, B; Strambi, S. Cross-correlation time-frequency analysis for multiple EMG signals in Parkinson's disease: a wavelet approach. *Medical Engineering and Physics*, 2003 25, 361-369.

Morrenhof, J; Abbink, H. Cross-correlation and cross-talk in surface electromyography. *Electromyography and Clinical Neurophysiology*, 1985 25, 73-79.

Nagata, K; Ando, K; Magatani, K; Yamada, M. Development of the hand motion recognition system based on surface EMG using suitable measurement channels for pattern recognition. In: André Dittmar, editor. *Proceedings of the 29th Annual International Conference of the IEEE EMBS*. Lyon, Flance: IEEE EMBS; 2007; 5214-5217.

Oksanen, A; Ylinen, JJ; Poyhonen, T; Anttila, P; Laimi, K; Hiekkanen, H; Salminen, JJ. Repeatability of electromyography and force measurements of the neck muscles in adolescents with and without headache. *Journal of Electromyography and Kinesiology*, 2007 17, 493-503.

Õunpuu, S; De Luca, PA; Bell, KJ; Davis, RB. Using surface electrodes for the evaluation of the rectus femoris, vastusmedialis and vastuslateralis muscles in children with cerebral palsy. *Gait and Posture*, 1997 5(3), 211-216.

Parker, P; Englehart, K; Hudgins, B. Myoelectric signal processing for control of powered limb prostheses. *Journal of Electromyography and Kinesiology*, 2006 16, 541-548.

Perry, J; Davis, B; Luciano, M. Quantifying muscle activity in non-ambulatory children with spastic cerebral palsy before and after selective dorsal rhizotomy. *Journal of Electromyography and Kinesiology*, 2001 11, 31-37.

Perry, J. Distal rectus femoris transfer. *Developmental Medicine and Child Neurology*, 1987 29(2), 153-8.

Prilutsky, B. Coordination of two-and one-joint muscles: functional consequences and implications for motor control. *Motor control*, 2000 4, 1 -44.

Psek, J; Cafarelli, E. Behavior of coactive muscles during fatigue. *Journal of Applied Physiology*, 1993 74, 170-5.

Pullman, S; Goodin, D; Marquinez, A;Tabbal, M; Rubin, M. Clinical utility of surface EMG. *Neurology*, 2000 55, 171-177.

Rau, G; Schulte, E; Disselhorst-Klug, C. From cell to movement: to what answers does EMG really contribute? *Journal of Electromyography and Kinesiology*, 2004 14, 611-617.

Ricken, A; Bennett, S; Savelsbergh, G. Coordination of reaching in children with spastic hemiparetic cerebral palsy under different task demands. *Motor Control*, 2005 9, 357-71.

Smith, M; Coppieters, M; Hodges, P. Is balance different in women with and without stress urinary incontinence? *Neurology Urodyn*, 2008 27, 71-78.

Solomonow, M; Baratta, R; Bernardi, M; Zhou, B; Lu, Y; Zhu, M; Acierno, S. Surface and wire EMG crosstalk in neighbouring muscles. *Journal of Electromyography and Kinesiology*, 1994 4(3), 131-142.

Staudenmann, D; Kingma, I; Stegeman, DF; van Dieen, JH. Towards optimal multi-channel EMG electrode configurations in muscle force estimation; a high density EMG study. *Journal of Electromyography and Kinesiology*, 2005 15,1-11.

Staudenmann, D; Daffertshoer, A; Kingma, I; Stegeman, D; van Dieën, J. Independent component analysis of high-density electromyography in muscle force estimation. *IEEE Transactions on Biomedical Engineering*, 2007 54, 751 – 754.

Staudenmann, D; Kingma, I; Daffertshoer, A; Stegeman, D; van Dieën, J. Improving EMG-based muscle force estimation by using a high-density EMG grid and principal component analysis. *IEEE Transactions on Biomedical Engineering*, 2006 53, 712-719.

Staudenmann, D; Stegeman, D; van Dieën, J. Methodological aspects of SEMG recordings for force estimation: A tutorial and review. *Journal of Electromyography and Kinesiology*, 2010 20, 375-387.

Sutherland, DH. Dynamic Electromyography by Age. In : Sutherland DH, Olshen RA, Biden EN, Wyatt MP, editors. *The Development of Mature Walking*. London: MacKeith Press; 1988; 154-162.

Sutherland, DH. The evolution of clinical gait analysis part 1: kinesiological EMG. *Gait and Posture*, 2001 14, 61-70.

Valkeinen, H; Ylinen, J; Malkia, E. Maximal force, force/time and activation/ coactivation characteristics of the neck muscles in extension and flexion in healthy men and women at different ages. *European Journal of Applied Physiology*, 2002 88, 247–54.

van Dieen, J; Cholewicki, J; Radebold, A. Trunk muscle recruitment patterns in patients with low back pain enhance the stability of the lumbar spine. *Occupational Health/ Ergonomics*, 2003 28, 834-841.

van Dijk, J; Blok, J; Lapatki, B; van Schaik, I; Zwarts, M; Stegeman, D. Motor unit number estimation using high-density surface electromyography. *Clinical Neurophysiology*, 2008 119, 33-42.

van Der Weel, FR; van Der Meer, ALH; Lee, DN. Influence of task on movement control in children with cerebral palsy: implications for research and therapy (in Dutch: Involed van taak op bewegingscontrol-ebijkinderen met cerebraalparese: implicatiesvooronderzoek en therapie). *Nederlands Tijdschriftvoor Fysiotherapier*, 1995 105, 138-44.

von Tscharner, V. Intensity analysis in time-frequency space of surface myoelectric signals by wavelets of specified resolution. *Journal of Electromyography and Kinesiology*, 2000 10, 433-445.

von Tscharner, V; Nigg, B. Point: spectral properties of the surface EMG can characterize/do not provide information about motor unit recruitment strategies and muscle fiber type. *Journal of Applied Physiology*, 2008105, 1671-3.

Wren, T; Do, K; Rethlefsen, S; Healy, B. Cross-correlation as a method for comparing dynamic electromyography signals during gait. *Journal of Biomechanics*, 2006 39, 2714-2718.

Yack, H. Techniques for clinical assessment of human movement. *Physical Therapy*, 1984 64,1821-1830.

Yang, J; Winter, D. Electromyographic amplitude normalizing methods, improving their sensitivity as diagnostic tools in gait analysis. *Archives of Physical Medicine and Rehabilitation*, 1984 65, 517-521.

Ylinen, JJ; Rezasoltanib, A; Julinc, MV; Virtapohjac, HA; Mälkiäc, EA. Reproducibility of isometric strength: measurement of neck muscles. *Clinical Biomechanics*, 1999 14(3), 217-219.

Ylinen, J; Salo, P; Nykänen, M; Kautiainen, H; Häkkinen, **A.** Decreased isometric neck strength in women with chronic neck pain and the repeatability of neck strength measurements. *Archives of Physical Medicine and Rehabilitation*, 2004 85(8), 1303-1308.

Young, CC; Rose, SE; Biden, EN. The effect of surface and internal electrodes on the gait of children with cerebral palsy, spastic diplegic type. *Journal of Orthopaedic Research*, 1989 7(5), 732-737.

Zwarts, M; Drost, G; Stegeman, D. Recent progress in the diagnostic use of surface EMG for neurological diseases. *Journal of Electromyography and Kinesiology*, 2000 10, 287-291.

Zwarts, M; Stegeman, D. Multichannel surface EMG: Basic aspects and clinical utility. *Muscle & Nerve*, 2003 28, 1-17.

In: Electromyography
Editor: Hiroki Takada

ISBN: 978-1- 62081-717-9

Chapter II

Clinical Trials with Surface Electromyography

Luciane Aparecida Pascucci Sande,
Luciane Fernanda Rodrigues Martinho Fernandes
and Marcia Souza Volpe
Physiotherapy Department at the Federal University of Triângulo Mineiro,
Minas Gerais, Brazil

Abstract

Studies using surface electromyography (EMG) as clinical and investigational instruments have expanded over the last few years and the presented results have contributed in different areas of knowledge. The area of rehabilitation may benefit from this technology, both as an assessment, assistance and monitoring of therapeutic treatments. Based on the literature new findings and looking for help in the decision-making in the clinical setting, the present chapter will show results of a pilot and complete studies involving subareas in the field of rehabilitation. *I)* The first part of this chapter presents excerpts of two published articles in Parkinson's disease (PD). As the main results of the first study, in which the sit-to-stand task was investigated, it can be listed: 1) the EMG sign was similar in subjects with moderate PD and healthy subjects; 2) both groups used co-activation patterns, nevertheless the magnitude of the PD group co-activation was considerably larger; 3) the use of verbal and visual cues seems to help start the movement in subjects with PD by the use of cerebellar-premotor cortex pathways, which are intact in this population. In a second study, with Parkinson's disease subjects, the multi-joint movements with reversal were explored, and the obtained results are: 1) there was a reduction of EMG activity and a simultaneous activation of antagonists in subjects with PD; 2) subjects with PD had difficulties in modulation the EMG activity during the different phases of the movement. Unlike the healthy subjects, the PD individuals presented an elevated level of EMG activity during the phases in which the muscles should demonstrate a reduced activity. However the problem is not that PD individuals have difficulty in reducing the EMG amount during acceleration of the limb towards the target, but the incapacity to keep a vigorous level of muscle activation capable of accelerating towards the target direction. *II)* In the second part of this chapter it is presented a preliminary study designed to evaluate the strategy to medial-lateral stability in ankle through EMG activity in different tasks in health subjects and in one subject with sprain. The results indicated: 1) fibularis brevis is an important medial-lateral stabilizer and need to be better investigated in EMG studies and also in the clinical setting; 2) in presence of a sprain, it was observed an important activity of tibialis anterior in all tasks, which might be avoided with some exercises and postural awareness; 3) it is important to know that the muscles in the contra lateral lower limb, are not activated as before the sprain. *III)* Finally, in the last part of the chapter, it is showed a possible use of EMG in the presence of pulmonary diseases. The aim of this pilot study was to evaluate the influence of forward leaning on inspiratory muscular activity and inspired tidal volume (V_T) during the performance of breathing exercises in patients with chronic obstructive pulmonary disease (COPD). The preliminary results are: 1) considering all four tested inspiratory muscular groups, electromyographic activity does not seem to be different between the two thoracic positions, forward leaning versus upright sitting, in COPD patients; 2) altering the thoracic position did not affect the mean inspired V_T in the healthy subject and in the COPD patients. The proposal is to continue the collects with healthy subjects and COPDs patients to better understand the effects of forward leaning on respiratory mechanics in patients with COPD. All these results offer new possibilities of studies and they also bring important messages that have to be incorporated in the clinical practice of a physiotherapist.

I) Electromyography in Parkinson's Disease

In a recent article untitled: *The effect of the restricted sit-to-stand task on biomechanical variables in subjects with and without parkinson's disease*, published in Journal of Electromyography and Kinesiology (JEK) we investigated the electromyographic activity in a very common daily life activity: the rising from a seated position. Another interesting issue that we explored was the differences between muscles activations patterns in subjects with Parkinson's disease and healthy subjects during the performance of complexes movements. The article was also published in JEK, with the title: *Multi-joint movements with reversal in Parkinson's disease: kinematics and electromyography*. Syntheses of the main comments and electromyographic results of referred articles will be presented below.

1) Sande de Souza, Luciane Aparecida Pascucci; Curtarelli, Mônica de Biagi; Mukherjee, Mukul; Dionísio, Valdeci Carlos. *The effect of the restricted sit-to-stand task on biomechanical variables in subjects with and without parkinson's disease.* Journal of Electromyography and Kinesiology, available online: 1 june 2011, *doi:10.1016/j.jelekin. 2011.04.007.*

Short Introduction

Rising from a seated position is a basic functional task, incorporated in daily life functions (Krajl et al., 1990; Reisman et al, 2002). Sit-to-stand has been identified as one of the most mechanically demanding motor tasks among activities of daily life, confirming the general acceptance of their effectiveness as indicators of the mobility level (Goulart & Valls-Solé, 1999; Hughes et al.,1996; Kerr et al., 1997; Mazzà et al., 2005).

During sit-to-stand, Parkinson's disease (PD) subjects demonstrate a large proportion of muscular co-contraction because they move slower (Bishop et al., 2005). A difficulty in initiating the movement could produce smaller horizontal velocity which could be caused by a deficit in recruiting muscles, such as the tibialis anterior (Bishop et al., 2005) and hip flexors (Mak et al., 2003). The slowness of the movement in the PD subjects may be associated with muscle weakness (Nogaki et al., 2001), especially in the muscles around the knee. The aim of this study was to compare the pattern of muscular activation during sit-to-stand in subjects with and without PD.

Methods: Electromyographic Measurements

Fifteen subjects voluntarily participated in the study (7 healthy subjects (NN group) and 8 subjects with Parkinson's disease (PD group)). For the subjects with Parkinson's disease, the mean duration of disease was 7.4 (±3.5) years. All the subjects with PD showed bilateral involvement with a great impairment on the right side and were classified as stage II or III in the Hoehn and Yahr scale. All PD subjects were medicated and undergoing physiotherapeutic treatment during the period of the tests. The tests were conducted in the morning after 12 hours of medication withdrawal All subjects signed a consent form approved by the University Office of Research Ethics.

The sit-to-stand task was done using a chair with adjustable height. The initial position of the subject was a comfortable sitting posture, maintaining about 70° of hip flexion and 60° of knee flexion. The shoulders were kept at 90 degrees of flexion to partially limit the trunk movements in the sagittal plane, as done for downward squatting (Cheron et al., 1997; Dionisio et al., 2008). Targets were determined for each subject based on their characteristic anthropometry and were positioned in front of the subjects on an acrylic board. The subjects were instructed to perform the sit-to-stand movement as fast as possible using the arm as reference, to achieve marker 1 in the beginning of the movement and marker 2 (target) at the end. The movement was visually guided and began after a verbal command: "prepare and go". Ten trials were performed after a period of training (3 trials).

The electromyographic (EMG) activities of the tibialis anterior (TA), soleus (SO), vastus medialis oblique (VMO), biceps femoris (BF) and erector spinae (ES) were recorded with bipolar surface DelSYS electrodes (model DE2.2L). The electrodes were fixed after the skin surface was shaved, abraded, and cleaned with alcohol. For the VMO, the electrode was placed on the muscle belly, along the direction of the fibers (about 54°) and 2 cm distal from the motor point (Bevilaqua-Grossi et al., 2004). To find the motor point, the subject was asked to perform an isometric contraction of the quadriceps so that the VMO activity could be observed. The electrode was then placed as close as possible to the retinaculum. For the other muscles, the electrodes were placed according to the guidelines of the SENIAM project (Surface ElectroMyoGraphy for the Non-Invasive Assessment of Muscles) from the Biomedical Health and Research Program (BIOMED II) of the European Union (Hermens et al., 2000). The EMG signals were amplified (x 2000), band-pass filtered (20-450 Hz) and recorded at 1000 Hz.

The EMG signals collected during the movements were rectified, filtered (low-pass at 20 Hz using a second-order Butterworth filter) and normalized to the averaged EMG signal recorded for the tested muscle during maximum voluntary isometric contraction (MVIC). The averaged EMG of the MVIC was calculated within the 500 to 1000 ms interval from the beginning of the isometric contraction.

The mean of EMG activities were calculated for each of the 4 phases which were based on the knee angular velocity: before the beginning of the movement (1), acceleration, (2) deceleration (3) and after the end of movement (4). Phase 1 was calculated for an interval of 100 milliseconds (ms) just before the knee velocity first achieved 5% of its peak, characterizing the pre-standup period. Phases 2 and 3 defined the acceleration and the deceleration time of the task, and included, respectively, the interval from the end of phase 1 to the time point where knee velocity achieved its peak and from the end of phase 2 to the time point where knee velocity returned to 5% of its peak. Phase 4 defined the time when the body remained at the target position, for a time interval of 100 ms, following the end of phase 3 (Dionisio et al., 2008).

STATISTICA for Windows (StatSoft, Inc., Tulsa, OK; version 5.0) was used for analysis. ANOVA with repeated measures design was used to test the effect of the groups and of the movement phases (1 to 4) on the dependent variable (EMG signals from the recorded muscles). A post-hoc comparison using the Tukey honest significant difference was conducted to test significant differences between specific phases. Alpha was set at 0.05.

Results and Discussion about EMG Data

For EMG activities the ANOVA did not reveal any effect of the group ($F_{(1,13)}$=0.00; p=0.95) for VMO, for TA, ($F_{(1,13)}$=1.61; p=0.22), for BF, ($F_{(1,13)}$=2.25; p=0.15), for SO, ($F_{(1,13)}$=3.78; p=0.07), or for ES, ($F_{(1,13)}$=1.53; p=0.23).

The behavior of the EMG activity was characteristic for each group. In the NN group, the TA and SO were co-activated to stabilize the ankle thereby allowing the movement of the knee and hip joints to be performed with stability and precision (Dionisio et al., 2008). The EMG activities of the BF, VMO and ES observed in this study were very important to counter the gravitational force (especially in the phases 2 and 3). The action of the BF is necessary to pull the pelvis and help with hip extension (Ohkoshi et al., 1991) during sit-to-stand. This is in agreement with a previous study (Goulart & Valls-Solé, 1999) which classified the muscles related with the task according to the functions exerted by them. TA and SO were considered postural muscles, while ES, quadriceps and hamstrings were considered the prime movers.

The results of the PD group showed differences in the amount of the EMG activity only in qualitative terms. The apparent increased co-activation in the PD group could be the result of either specific Parkinsonian characteristics or trunk restriction or both.

Muscular co-activation patterns have been shown during several activities in subjects with PD (Bishop et al., 2005; Horak et al., 1992). Co-activation is believed to have occurred because the antagonist muscles were activated at larger than normal magnitudes and at shorter-than-normal latencies (Dimitrova et al., 2004). Co-activation may also serve as a default strategy to defend against potential perturbations. Both groups used co-activation, although, the magnitude of the PD group co-activation was considerably larger. It seems that they were using *coactive stiffening*, which reflects in an increased co-activation of postural muscle bursts, increased stiffness of inherent passive elastic muscle elements and increased stiffness from increased background tonic activity (Dimitrova et al, 2004).

Finally, some characteristics of motor responses are relatively unaffected by Parkinson´s disease, perhaps because externally triggered movements can also be controlled via extrastriatal pathways (Horak et al., 1992). The present experiment used verbal and visual cues as external stimulus to trigger the movement, which utilizes cerebellar-premotor cortex pathways. Such pathways may be intact in subjects with PD. This may be a reason why the subjects with PD did not show substantial differences in comparison to the healthy controls. Several studies have explored the utility of such external cues in a clinical setting (Rubinstein et al., 2002; Suteerawattananon et al., 2004; Rochester et al., 2005).

References

Bevilaqua-Grossi, D., Pedro, V. M. & Bérzin F. (2004). Análise funcional dos estabilizadores patelares. *Acta Ortop Bras*, *12*, 99-104.

Bishop, M., Brunt, D., Pathare, N., Ko, M. & Marjama-Lyons, J. (2005). Changes in distal muscle timing may contribute to slowness during sit to stand in Parkinson's disease. *Clin Biomech (Bristol, Avon)*, *20*, 112-7.

Cheron, G., Bengoetxea, A., Pozzo, T., Bourgeois, M. & Draye, J. P. (1997). Evidence of a preprogrammed deactivation of the hamstring muscles for triggering rapid changes of posture in humans. *Electroenceph Clin Neurophysiol*, *105*, 58-71.

Dimitrova, D., Horak, F. B. & Nutt, J. G. (2004). Postural muscle responses to multidirectional translations in patients with Parkinson's disease. *J Neurophysiol*, *91*, 489-01.

Dionisio, V. C., Almeida, G. L., Duarte, M. & Hirata, R. P. (2008). Kinematic, Kinetic and EMG Patterns during Downward Squatting. *J Electromyogr Kinesiol*, *18,* 134-43.

Goulart, F. R. & Valls-Solé, J. (1999). Patterned electromyographic activity in the sit-to-stand movement. *Clin Neurophysiol*, *110*, 1634-40.

Hermens, H. J., Freriks, B., Disselhorst-Klug, C. & Rau, G. (2000). Development of recommendations for SEMG sensors and sensor placement procedures. *J Electromyogr Kinesiol*, *10*, 361-74.

Horak, F. B., Nutt, J. & Nashner, L. M. (1992). Postural inflexibility in Parkinsonian subjects. *J Neurol Sci*, *111*, 46-58.

Hughes, M. A., Myers, B. S. & Schenkman, M. L. (1996). The role of strength in rising from a chair in the functionally impaired elderly. *J Biomech*, *29*, 1509-13.

Kerr, K. M., White, J. A., Barr, D. A. & Mollan, R. A. (1997). Analysis of the sit-stand-sit movement cycle in normal subjects. *Clin Biomech (Bristol, Avon)*, *12*, 236-45.

Krajl, A., Jaeger, R. J. & Munih, M. (1990). Analysis of standing up and sitting down in humans: definitions and normative data presentation. *J Biomech*, *23*, 1123-38.

Mak, M. K., Levin, O., Mizrahi, J. & Hui-Chan, C. W. (2003). Joint torques during sit-to-stand in healthy subjects and people with Parkinson's disease. *Clin Biomech (Bristol, Avon)*, *18*, 197-06.

Mazzà, C., Zok, M. & Croce, U. D. (2005). Sequencing sit-to-stand and upright posture for mobility limitation assessment: determination of the timing of the task phases from force platform data. *Gait & Posture*, *21*, 425-31.

Nogaki, H., Kakinuma, S. & Morimatsu, M. (2001). Muscle weakness in Parkinson's disease: a follow-up study. Parkinsonism *Relat Disord*, *8*, 57-62.

Ohkoshi, Y., Yasuda, K., Kaneda, K., Wada, T. & Yamanaka M. (1991). Biomechanical analysis of rehabilitation in the standing position. *Am J Sports Med*, *19*, 605-7.

Ramsey, V. K., Miszko, T. A. & Horvat, M. (2004). Muscle activation and force production in Parkinson's patients during sit to stand transfers. *Clin Biomech (Bristol, Avon)*, *19*, 377-84.

Reisman, D. S., Scholz, J. P. & Schoner, G. (2002). Differential joint coordination in the tasks of standing up and sitting down. *J Electromyogr Kinesiol*,*12*, 493-05.

Rochester, L., Hetherington, V., Jones, D., Nieuwboer, A., Willems, A., Kwakkel, G. & Van Wegen, E. (2005). The Effect of external rhythmic cues (auditory and visual) on walking during a functional task in homes of people with Parkinson's disease. *Arch Phys Med Rehabil*, *86*, 999-1006.

Rubinstein, T. C., Giladi, N. & Hausdorff, J. M. (2002). The power of cueing to circumvent dopamine deficits: A review of physical therapy treatment of gait disturbances in Parkinson's disease. *Mov Disord*, *17*, 1148-60.

Seidler, R. D., Alberts, J. L. & Stelmach, G. E. (2001). Multijoint movement control in Parkinson's disease. *Exp Brain Res*, *140*, 335-44.

Suteerawattananon, M., Morris, G. S., Etnyre, B. R., Jankovic, J. & Protas E. J. (2004). Effects of visual and auditory cues on gait in individuals with Parkinson's disease. *J Neurol Sci*, *219*, 63-69.

2) Sande de Souza, Luciane Aparecida Pascucci; Dionísio, Valdeci Carlos; Almeida, Gil Lúcio . *Multi-joint movements with reversal in Parkinson s disease: Kinematics and electromyography.* Journal of Electromyography and Kinesiology, v. 21, p. 376-383, 2010.

Short Introduction

Some authors showed that subjects with Parkinson's disease (PD) had great difficulty in performing multi-joint movements involving some degrees of freedom (Teulings et al., 1997; Alberts et al., 1998; Poizner et al., 1998). Teulings et al. (1997) observed that Parkinson's subjects had coordination problems during simultaneous finger movements. Also, Alberts et al. (1998) suggested that PD subjects have difficulty in specifying and regulating multiple task-level degrees of freedom independently. It has often been reported that PD subjects experience difficulties in switching from one movement to another (Weiss et al., 1997).

According to Berardelli et al. (2001), the slowness of single-joint movements observed in PD subjects is caused by problems in recruiting the appropriate level of muscle force sufficiently fast. If any additional complexity is added to a simple movement, such slowness becomes more evident. The PD subjects may be trying to compensate for lack of basal ganglia input by devoting more resources to each single task they perform. When more than one task is required, this becomes a limiting factor. In the same way, Hallet and Khoshbin (1980) observed that ballistic movements are accompanied by a triphasic electromyographic (EMG) pattern. Such a pattern is present in PD subjects, but the first agonist burst is small.

Therefore, the PD subjects often add further bursts of EMG to the pattern in order to achieve enough force to move the limb to the required end position.

These findings reveal the difficulty PD subjects have during the performance of fast ballistic movements, because they cannot inject a large enough initial burst of EMG activity. They achieve the movement by a repetitive series of small agonist bursts (Marsden, 1982; Hallett and Koshbin, 1980; Day et al., 1984; Berardelli et al., 1986; Berardelli et al., 1996, Pfann et al., 2001).

Most studies of multi-joint arm movements in subjects with PD have reported kinematics and even kinetics (Alberts et al., 2000; Phillips et al., 1994; Poizner et al., 2000; Rand et al., 2002), but no muscle activities. Only Farley et al. (2004) extended the findings of single joint studies to multi-joint movements. They showed that PD subjects produced several burst abnormalities, such as deficits in initial agonist burst amplitude and duration at fast and slow speeds.

Based on such results, a hypothesis raised was whether the slowness of movements would be generated by a reduction in EMG activity or had a lack of modulation in the phases of acceleration and deceleration during the reach-to-grasp movements and return to the initial position.

Methods: Electromyographic Measurements

Nine healthy subjects with mean age of 66 ± 8.52 and ten PD subjects (five men and five women) older than 50 years (66.2 ± 10.0) were tested according to protocols approved by the Research Ethics Committee of the State University of Campinas – UNICAMP, and all subjects assigned an informed consent form. The PD subjects had been diagnosed (Gelb et al., 1999) with bilateral or unilateral idiopathic Parkinson's disease, but none of them had other neurological disease determined by exam or history as well as other lesion, disorder, or use of medication that could intervene with their motor function. These data were obtained by a neurologist's evaluation. Healthy and PD subjects were sedentary and right-handed, with the tests being conducted on their right arm. The tests were conducted during the morning because in this part of the day the PD individuals were in the off period (about 12 hours after the last ingestion of medication) (Pffan et al., 2001, Robichaud et al., 2002).

After calculating a coordinate system on an acrylic board each subject performed reversal movements in the sagittal plane, involving elbow and shoulder excursion regarding three target locations, with wrist and hand immobilized by a thermoplastic splint (Sande de Souza et al., 2009). At the initial position, shoulder was at zero degree of flexion (upper arm aligned with the trunk) and elbow at 45° (external angle). Each of the three targets were placed in such a way that the elbow joint was at full extension (45°), combined with three angular excursions of the shoulder joint (30°, 60° or 90° of flexion, which increased in a counterclockwise direction). However, it is important to note that there was no elbow constraint. Thus, the linear distance of each target was different for each subject due to individual anthropometric differences. The target location was defined with a small ball of cotton placed on the acrylic board. The subjects were instructed to perform the task (go to the target and return to the initial position) "as fast and as accurately as possible". The presentation sequence of target locations was randomized for each subject, with the subjects performing 15 attempts for each target although only the last 10 ones were recorded.

Bipolar active surface electrodes (model DE2.2L, DelSYS Inc., Boston, MA, USA) were placed on the following muscles of the right upper limb: anterior deltoid, posterior deltoid, biceps brachialis (long head), and triceps brachialis (lateral head) after the skin surface was shaved, abraded, and cleaned with alcohol. The EMG signals were amplified (x 2000), band-pass filtered (20-450 Hz), and recorded. These data were digitized at 12 bits and collected by an IBM computer at 1000 Hz.

The electromyographic data were processed offline using a Matlab software (Math Works Inc., version 6.0). In this routine, the movement was divided into two phases: the reaching phase, when the subject moves towards the target, and the return phase, when the subject returns towards the initial position. Both reaching and the returning phases were further divided: the acceleration and deceleration phases towards and from the target, respectively. Five landmarks of the fingertip speed defined each of the four movement phases. Line 1 demarcates the time point when fingertip speed first exceeded 5% of its peak value; line 2, when it first achieved its peak; line 3, when it returned to the smallest value at the target (reversal time); line 4, when it achieved its second peak, and finally; line 5, when it returned for the third time to 5% of its value.

Thus, the four movement phases were defined as: I) Acceleration towards the target (from line 1 to line 2); II) deceleration towards the target (line 2 to line 3); III) acceleration from the target to the initial position (line 3 to 4); and IV) deceleration from the target to the initial position (line 4 to 5).

The electromyographic signs (EMG) were rectified and filtered, and the integrals were normalized by the duration time of them. So, the result was a mean of the electrical activity regarding these muscles during the period of measured integral. The same approach was used by Pffan et al. (2001) in a previous study, who also investigated healthy and PD subjects.

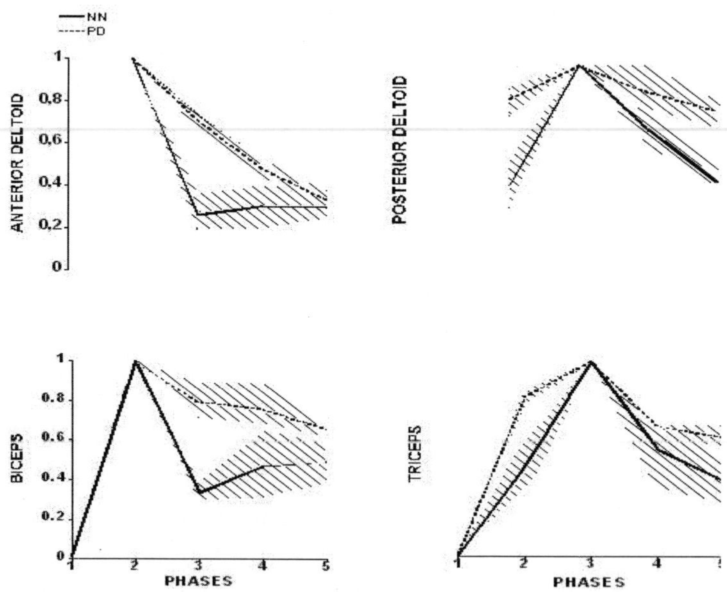

Figure 1. Index of electromyographic activity (EMG) for each muscle. X-axis: phase 1 (basal activity), phases 2-5 (the four phases of the linear speed). The thick lines: means of the three target distances (NN:full line, SP:dashed line). Shaded lines: the limit values obtained.

It is worth mentioning that EMG data normalization by maximal voluntary contraction (MVC) cannot be conducted because of the maximum slow values of PD population. Such normalization could generate wrong values. To solve this problem, it was created an index from the maximum values of EMG activity generated in each interval of linear speed. So, the observed activities in the other phases are percentage values for this index.

In order to evaluate effect of the groups, target locations (three targets), and movement direction (towards and from the target), it was used two-way factorial ANOVA with repeated measures: [group (NN and PD) X muscles (each muscle activity separately in each interval)]. As a *post hoc* test, we used the least-significant difference (LSD) method. Data were analyzed in a personal computer using the statistical software Statistica for Windows (Statsoft, Inc. version 5.0). For all evaluations, the significance level (α) was set at 0.05.

Results about EMG Data

As mentioned before, we will present the index from maximum values of EMG activity generated in each interval of linear speed. The observed activities in the other phases are percentage values for this index (Figure 1).

With regard to the shoulder, PD subjects are different from the healthy subjects in some aspects: they always generated a lower level of muscle activity (anterior deltoid and biceps activity); in the phase 2, the action of anterior deltoid was high and the posterior deltoid activity was low for the movement required.

By analyzing the elbow joint, it was observed in phase 1 that the high biceps activity was influenced by the distance ($F_{(2,34)}$= 12,26; p=0.00). In phase 2, when the subjects decelerate towards the target direction, one can observe the triceps action clearly, followed by a more prominent activity of the biceps during phase 3. During the phase 4, the pattern observed in phase 1 tends to repeat itself. The PD subjects demonstrated some difficult in coordinating this balance between biceps and triceps activation.

The findings have revealed that PD subjects have difficulty in modulating the muscle bursts, and this temporal modulation is negatively affected by the increase in the movement distance (Figure 1). ANOVAs were conducted for all muscles and the results showed statistically significant differences between groups, distances and phases of linear speed regarding all the phases, except for posterior deltoid. The following values were obtained for anterior deltoid: group ($F_{(1,17)}$=9.46; p=0.00), distance ($F_{(2,34)}$=99.93; p=0.00) and phases ($F_{(3,51)}$ 42.47; p=0.00); for posterior deltoid: group ($F_{(1,17)}$=26.18; p=0.00), distance ($F_{(2,34)}$=17.84 p=0.00) and phases ($F_{(3,51)}$=1.04; p=0.38); for biceps: group ($F_{(1,17)}$=5.01; p=0.03), distance ($F_{(2,34)}$= 25.29; p=0.00) and phases ($F_{(3,51)}$=8.44; p=0.00); and for triceps: group ($F_{(1,17)}$=3.92; p=0.05), distance ($F_{(2,34)}$=24.10; p=0.00) and phases ($F_{(3,51)}$=5.74; p=0.00).

Overall, all the subjects exhibited a similar pattern that had been previously observed as well, that is, a high activity of anterior deltoid and biceps in phase 1 and more prominent activities of posterior deltoid and triceps in phases 2 and 3. Such activities are in accordance with the task, but it is important to note that PD subjects always presented a tendency to recruit several muscles in all phases at the same time, even the antagonists.

Discussion about EMG Data

The hypothesis was confirmed by the movement slowness developed by PD subjects with the reduction of EMG activity associated with a simultaneous activation of antagonists. In addition, PD individuals presented difficulties in modulating the EMG activity during each phase of the movement. Such findings determined a typical basal ganglia function for the control of the amount of EMG activity and agonist-antagonist relation as well.

For movements with reversal, healthy individuals demonstrate a capacity to modulate the EMG activity in accordance with the mechanical demands of the task in accordance with the mechanical demands of the task (Gottlieb, 1998). Such capacity is impaired in PD subjects, since they presented a reduction in the amount of EMG agonist and antagonist activities compared to healthy subjects. This EMG activity reduction in PD subjects was also found in single-joint movements without (Hallet and Khoshbin, 1980; Robichaud et al., 2002; Berardelli et al., 1996) and with reversal (Pffan et al., 2001; Pffan et al., 2004; Seidler et al., 2001).

Qualitative changes in the EMG patterns, characterized by a simultaneous activation of agonist and antagonist muscles are described to the PD subjects during pointing and reversal movements (Seidler et al., 2001; Pfann et al., 2001; Pfann et al., 2004). The data presented here corroborate these observations (Figure 1).

During the movements with reversal in healthy subjects, a first burst of EMG activity occurs in the muscles, which initially accelerates the limb towards the target direction (DA and BIC, see phase 2 in Figure 1). In the subsequent phases (reach deceleration, acceleration and deceleration of the return movement), the amount of activity of these muscles is abruptly reduced (Figure 1). Deceleration of the limb towards the target is abruptly increased in the EMG activity of the antagonist muscles (DP and TRI), which decelerate the limb movement from the target, revert the movement direction, and accelerate the return of the limb to its initial position (see phase 3, Figure 1). The quantity of this antagonist activity is reduced abruptly in other phases of the movement. In other words, for movements with reversal, healthy subjects modulate the EMG activity according to the mechanic demands of the task. Such findings only confirm what was observed by Almeida et al. (2005).

Unlike the healthy subjects, the PD individuals presented an elevated level of EMG activity during the phases in which the muscles should demonstrate a reduced activity (Figure 1). Although EMG activities of PD subjects were high during the phases they should be reduced, both groups did not turn off completely the muscles during all the movement phases (Figure 1). This activation of agonist and antagonist muscles is necessary to preserve the joint stability during the movement performance (Bazzucchi et al., 2006). Also, this activation could be related to the muscle stiffness presented in PD. Dimitrova et al. (2004) mention that PD subjects use coactive stiffening, which leads to increases in co-activation of postural muscle bursts, stiffness of inherent passive elastic muscle elements, and background tonic activity.

So, it seems that the problem is not that PD individuals have difficulty in reducing the EMG amount during acceleration of the limb towards the target, but the incapacity to keep a vigorous level of muscle activation capable of accelerating towards the target direction. This conclusion is in accordance with the findings of Seidler et al., 2001; Pfann et al., 2001; Pfann et al., 2004.

Several authors assign the PD subjects' difficulty in keeping an elevated level of agonist EMG activity to the basal ganglia impairment (Marsden, 1982; Day et al. 1984; Berardelli et al., 1986). The reduction of the agonist EMG activity during CVMs corroborates the study by Corcos et al. (1996), which might also reveal a decrease in excitatory projections of basal ganglia in the primary motor cortex (Marsden, 1982).

So, the EMG data described here confirm the hypothesis that muscle activity is reduced in PD subjects as they tend to adopt a co-activation pattern in several movement phases.

References

Alberts, J. L., Saling, M., Adler, C. H. & Stelmach, G. E. (2000). Disruptions in the reach-to grasp actions of Parkinson's patients. *Exp Brain Res*, *134*, 353–62.

Alberts, J. L., Tresilian, J. R. & Stelmach, G. E. (1998). The co-ordination and phasing of a bilateral prehension task. The influence of Parkinson's disease. *Brain*, *121(4)*, 725–42.

Almeida, G. L., Freitas, S. M. & Marconi, N. F. (2005). Coupling between muscle activities and muscle torques during horizontal-planar arm movements with direction reversal. *J Electromyogr Kinesiol*, *16(3)*, 303–11.

Bazzucchi, L., Sbriccoli, P., Marzattinocci, G. & Felici, F. (2006). Coactivation of the elbow antagonist muscles is not affected by the speed of movement in isokinetic exercise. *Muscle Nerve*, *33*, 191–9.

Berardelli, A., Dick, J. P., Rothwell, J. C., Day, B. L. & Marsden, C. D. (1986). Scaling of the size of the first agonist EMG burst during rapid wrist movements in patients with Parkinson's disease. *J Neurol Neurosurg Psychiatr*, *49(11)*, 1273–9.

Berardelli, A., Hallett, M., Rothwell, J. C., Agostino, R., Manfredi, M., Thompson P.D., & Marsden, C. D. (1996). Single-joint rapid arm movements in normal subjects and in patients with motor disorders. *Brain*, *119*, 661–74.

Berardelli, A., Rothwell, J. C., Thompson, P. D. & Hallett, M. (2001). Pathophysiology of bradykinesia in Parkinson's disease. *Brain*, *124(11)*, 2131–46.

Corcos, D. M., Chen, C. M., Quinn, N. P., McAuley, J. & Rothwell, J. C. (1996). Strength in Parkinson's disease: relationship to rate of force generation and clinical status. *Ann Neurol*, *39(1)*, 79–88.

Day, B. L., Dick, J. P. R. & Marsden, C. D. (1984). Patients with Parkinson's can employ a predictive motor strategy. *J Neurol Neurosurg Psychiatr*, *47*, 1299–306.

Dimitrova, D., Horak, F. B. & Nutt, J. G. (2004). Postural muscle responses to multidirectional translations in patients with Parkinson's disease. *J Neurophysiol*, *91(1)*, 489–501.

Farley, B. G., Sherman, S. & Koshland, G. F. (2004). Shoulder muscle activity in Parkinson's disease during multijoint arm movements across a range of speeds. *Exp Brain Res*, *154(2)*, 160–75.

Gelb, D. J., Oliver, E. & Gilman, S. (1999). Diagnosis criteria for Parkinson disease. *Arch Neurol*, *56*, 33–9.

Hallet, M. & Khoshbin, S. (1980). A physiological mechanism of bradykinesia. *Brain*, *103*, 301–4.

Hermens, H. J., Freriks, B., Disselhorst-Klug, C. & Rau, G. (2000). Development of recommendations for SEMG sensors and sensor placement procedures. *J Electromyogr Kinesiol*, *10*, 361–74.

Pfann, K. D., Buchman, A. S., Comella, C. L. & Corcos, D. M. (2001). Control of movement distance in Parkinson's disease. *Mov Disord*, *16(6)*, 1048–65.

Pfann, K. D., Robichaud, J. A., Gottlieb, G. L., Comella, C. L., Brandabur, M. & Corcos, D.M. (2004). Muscle activation patterns in point-to-point and reversal movements in healthy, older subjects and in subjects with Parkinson's disease. *Exp Brain Res*, *157(1)*, 67–78.

Phillips, J. G., Martin, K. E., Bradshaw, J. L. & Iansek, R. (1994). Could bradykinesia in Parkinson's disease simply be compensation? *J Neurol*, *241(7)*, 439–47.

Poizner, H., Feldman, A. G., Levin, M. F., Berkinblit, M. B., Hening, W. A., Patel, A. & Adamovich, S. V. (2000). The timing of arm-trunk coordination is deficient and vision-dependent in Parkinson's patients during reaching movements. *Exp Brain Res*, *133(3)*, 279–92.

Poizner, H., Fookson, O. I., Berkinblit, M. B., Hening, W., Feldman, G. & Adamovich, S. (1998). Pointing to remembered targets in 3D space in Parkinson´ s disease. *Motor Control*, *2*, 251–77.

Rand, M. K., Van Gemmert, A. W. & Stelmach, G. E. (2002). Segment difficulty in two-stroke movements in patients with Parkinson's disease. *Exp Brain Res*, *143(3)*, 383–93.

Robichaud, J. A., Pfann, K. D., Comella, C. L. & Corcos, D. M. (2002). Effect of medication on EMG patterns in individuals with Parkinson's disease. *Mov Disord*, *17(5)*, 950–60.

Sande de Souza, L. A. P., Dionísio, V. C., Lerena, M. A., Marconi, N. F. & Almeida, G. L. (2009). The linear covariance between joint muscle torques is not a generalized principle. *J Electromyogr Kinesiol*, *19(3)*, 171–9.

Seidler, R. D., Alberts, J. L. & Stelmach, G. E. (2001). Multijoint movement control in Parkinson's disease. *Exp Brain Res*, *140*, 335–44.

Teulings, H. L., Contreras-Vidal, J. L., Stelmach, G. E. & Adler, C. H. (1997). Parkinsonism reduced coordination of fingers, wrist, and arm in fine motor control. *Exp Neurol*, *146*, 159–70.

Weiss, P., Stelmach, G. E. & Hefter, H. (1997). Programming of a movement sequence in Parkinson's disease. *Brain*, *120(1)*, 91–102.

II) Electromyography in the Analysis of Lateral Ankle Stability

Introduction

The most common complication after ankle sprain is functional instability (FI). It is defined as clinical presence of instability complaints, with no evidence of anatomic lesions of ligaments' system (Gerber et al., 1998; Hertel, 2000; Konradsen and Ravn, 1991). However when there is objectively a ligament system unable due to joint flatness, assessed through functional-clinical tests, it receives the name of mechanical instability (Gerber et al, 1998;

Hals et al, 2000;. Hertel, 2000). Usually, FI pathogenesis may be considered multifactorial, envolving mechanic, muscle and sensory motor factors (Konradsen and Magnusson, 2000).

The main factors related to functional instability are alteration in activities (Konradsen e Ravn, 1991; Lofvenberg et al, 1995; Safran et al., 1999) and latency (Pacheco et al., 2005; Johson and Johson, 1993) of fibular muscles. However the analysis of relation between activities of agonist and antagonist muscles might reveal new information about instability.

Even though muscle activity from ankle has been widely studied in individuals with instability, most of biomechanical studies have evaluated response of locomotor apparatus under extreme controlled conditions, through simulated movements of the injury mechanism (Myers et al., 2003; Osborne et al., 2001; Vaes et al., 2001), not considering real or daily situations in bipedal and unipedal support as proposed in this study. Besides, some studies are focused in the analysis of athlete's instability (Suda et al., 2009; Pacheco et al., 2005; Santilli et al., 2005; Delahunt et al., 2006; Delahunt et al., 2010), whose neuromuscular responses are different from untrained individuals.

Bases on previously cited articles the following hypotheses were defined: 1) There is difference between muscle activation considering agonist and antagonists of ankle inversion; 2) There is difference between activation on each muscle in different daily tasks; 3) There's no difference between sides in health subjects; 4) There's difference in the neuromuscular activation pattern in patients with sprain.

In this way the aim in this chapter was to evaluate if the methodology used was sensitive in verifying differences in activies and to evaluate the strategy to medial-lateral stability in ankle through electromyographic activity of the muscles tibialis anterior, fibularis longus and fibularis brevis while performing different tasks in one subject with sprain and in healthy subjects.

Material and Methods

Seven volunteers (four men and three women), academics, mean age of 20 (±2,0) years old were evaluated. To select the volunteers, the inclusion criteria were: absence of joint or muscular lesion in the inferior limbs, muscle-skeletal pain, rheumatologic or vestibular disease. The same evaluation was performed in a 27-year old patient with diagnosis of sprain in inversion in right ankle. All subjects signed an informed consent and the project was approved by the Committee of Ethics and Research of the Federal University of Triângulo Mineiro, protocol n° 1470/09. The research was conducted in the Laboratory of Human Movement Analysis, in the city of Uberaba/MG – Brazil.

To perform electromyographic analysis skin was shaved and higienized with alcohol 70% and positioning of surface electrodes followed instructions by the SENIAM protocol (*Surface Electromyography for the Non-invasive Assessment of Muscles*). The electrodes were positioned in the muscles: tibialis anterior (TA), fibularis longus (FL) and fibularis brevis (FB) (Hermens et al., 2000).

The volunteers and the patient performed 4 tasks of maintained postures with bipodal (T1), tiptoe (T2), unipodal right (T3) and left unipodal (T4). While performing such tasks, the electromyographic sign of the 3 muscles were collected bilaterally and simultaneously, for 3 seconds. Also the electromyographic sign was collected during maximum voluntary isometric contraction (MVIC) of each muscle.

The electromyographic activity of the muscles was registered on the electromyograph EMG Systems of Brasil®, with 6 electromyographic channels, pass-band of 20 to 500 Hz, with common rejection mode > 120 dB, entry impedance > 10 MOhms and 100x gain in the sign conditioner and 20x in passive bipolar electrode, totalizing 2000x. The electrodes used were with Ag/AgCl, in a self-adhesive disc form with gel and 1 cm of diameter. The electromyographic sign was collected and then filtered. The values of sign amplitude were represented in a root mean square (RMS). The electromyographic values of each muscle were normalized through the ratio between RMS value and maximum value obtained during MVIC, of each muscle in each task, according to equation 1.

$$EMG_n\,[UA] = \frac{RMS\,[UA]}{Máximo\ CIVM\,[\mu V]} \qquad (1)$$

EMGn = normalized data of electromyographic activity; RMS = root mean square; Maximum MVIC = maximum value obtained in MVIC; MVIC = maximum voluntary isometric contraction; UA = Random unity; µV = micro volt

After calculating EMG it was created an index based on the maximum value of electromyographic activity in the 3 muscles, for each task. It was considered the value of 100% for the muscle with higher activity and the others were considered as percentage values of this index.

Results

Muscle activity was presented in the form of an index for a better visualization of the activation pattern. In this analysis it was considered the value of 100% for the muscle with greater activity and the others as a percentage value of this index (Figure 2).

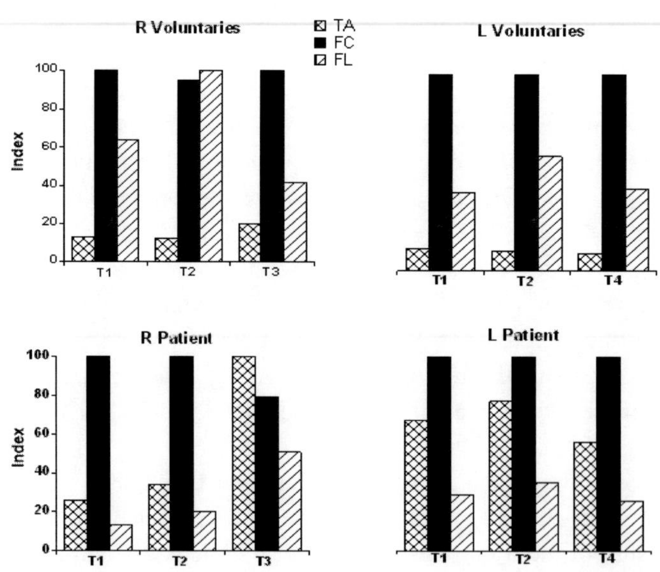

Figure 2. Index of muscle activity of volunteers and patient with sprain while performing the tasks.

In the analysis of activation patterns the sequence from greater to lesser electromyographic activation in patient was FB-TA-FL for all tasks in the left side and for tasks 1 and 2 in right side, while in task 3 it was TA-FB-FL. In the volunteers the sequence was FB-FL-TA for tasks 1 and 3 in right side and for all tasks on left side.

Discussion

This chapter complements literature about muscle actions that stabilize joint in a medial-lateral way, it also adds important information when exploring daily situations such as bipodal simple support, connected to orthostatic postural control, tiptoe and unipodal support. It also highlights the need to evaluate activities from fibularis brevis muscle, still under discussed in literature.

On regards to hypothesis described it was observed that in the index analysis there is a change in the muscle activation, considering health subjects and sprain patients. This chapter detaches the electromyographic activity from FB which is still few discussed in literature (Konradsen et al., 1998; Johnson and Johnson, 1993; Pacheco et al., 2005). In these cases the most analyzed muscles through surface electromyography are fibularis brevis, tibialis anterior and gastrocnemius, and activity from lateral component is limited to muscle fibularis longus (Palmieri-Smith and Hopkins, 2009; Eachaute et al., 2009; Vaes et al., 2002; Santili et al., 2005; Suda et al., 2009).

Higher activity from fibularis brevis in our study might be due to its predominance in the eversion of the foot (Kapandji, 2008). This suggests that fibularis brevis is a more eversor muscle than the fibularis longus. It participates in pronation of anterior part of the foot, enhancing extern metatarsal radius. In this last action, fibularis longus and extensor digitorum common reinforce it.

It is interesting to investigate the magnitude of electromyographic activity from inversors and eversors in individuals with functional instability. In this study, electromyographic analysis was sensitive in detecting differences in muscle activities of lateral stabilizers in the patient with sprain when compared to the injured side with the other and the health subjects.

Ankle sprains occurs during activities of daily living, however much researches about ankle sprain investigated muscle responses in individuals with and without ankle instability in extremely controlled situations, simulating the mechanism of lesion in sudden inversion of foot (Suda et al., 2009; Pacheco et al., 2005; Johnson and Jonhson, 1993).

In bipedal and unipedal support (Tasks 1,3 and 4) that involve control of erect posture, ankle strategy and muscle synergy of hip, knee and ankle are among the first patterns identified in anterior-posterior stability. Ankle strategy recovers stability position of the center of mass and requires full range of movement and muscle strength of ankle. Alternatives strategies are used to recover medial-lateral stability (Shumway-Cook and Woollacott, 2007). In the inferior limb medial-lateral movement is extremely reduced in ankle and knee joints, hip joint is the main used to recover medial-lateral stability (Rozendal, 1986; Day et al., 1993). For this last, when bilateral base of support is smaller than 8 cm there is an ankle movement to control this stability, but when it is higher, such movement is minimal. In this study, since the focus was the ankle, bilateral base of support was smaller than 8 cm, and proximal muscles of the inferior limb weren't explored.

According to Horak and Nashner (1986) health subject can rapidly substitute one postural strategy of movement for another, in other words, we are constantly modeling the amplitudes of postural responses. The same way, with repetitive exposition to a determined postural task, individuals refine the characteristics to optimize a task generating higher efficacy (Shumway-Cook and Woollacott, 2007; Moore et al., 1988). Such behavior can be observed in the variability of muscle responses in health subjects investigated in this study.

Even neuromuscular control is intact, in cases of muscle-skeletal alterations such as restriction of movement, changes in structure, muscle function and also alterations in production of strength; it might occur important restrictions in posture. Therefore, muscle-skeletal alterations may contribute to inability of maintenance of ideal alignment of body segments in the vertical position, demanding an excessive strength to fight the effects of gravity and maintain erect posture (Shumway-Cook and Wolollacott, 2007).

Based on these thoughts it is possible to highlight the high values of electromyographic activity of TA and FB associated with a smaller activation of FL in the patient with sprain, compared to health subjects. This reasoning supports the higher values found for the activation of TA and FB, and lower activation of FL, in the sprain patient compared to the normal individuals. There was similar alteration in the pattern of activation on the lesion side of the patient, with increased activation of TA and reduced activation of FB during the right side unipodal support task. An important point is to emphasize the activation of the three muscles on the side of the sprain, compared to both the opposite side. This seems to indicate that the amplitude and sequence of activations can change, as a compensatory defense mechanism. The data indicate that muscle activation can be bilaterally compromised following an acute lateral sprain of the ankle. This result is partially in agreement with the findings of a review and meta-analysis of bilateral equilibrium deficits following trauma to the ankle (Wikstrom et al., 2010). The same recommendations made by those authors can therefore be adapted for the results of the present work: 1) Following a sprain, the side not involved in the lesion should not be used as a reference for normal muscle activation; 2) patients with sprain should be submitted to fitness training for activation of the muscles of both lower limbs

This way, there is the modification in the pattern of contra lateral activation to the lesion: there is an increase in the activity of TA, but reduction in activity of FB. This seems to indicate that, temporarily, as a mechanism of compensation and defense, amplitudes and sequence of activations modify. Data reveal that muscle activity might be bilaterally impaired after a lateral ankle sprain. This result confirms findings from a review and meta analysis about bilateral balance deficits after ankle trauma (Wikstrom et al., 2010). This way, same recommendations from these authors can be adapted to the results of the present study: 1) after an ankle sprain, the non injured side should not be used as reference of normal muscle activity; 2) patients with sprain must be submitted to a practice of adequation of muscle activation in both inferior limbs. This practice is supported by the fact that neural adaptations that occur during balance reeducation happen in multiple places in the CNS (Wikstrom et al., 2010).

Present results also indicate that facing the injury, there are compensatory mechanisms that try to provide certain stability to ankle, among them the increase of activity of TA and FB can be highlighted. However Blackburn, Hirth and Guskiewicz, 2003 also observed increase in the activity of FL, that seemed to be connected to training. Is this increase caused by specific strengthening ou would it be fair to justify that it is a pattern of response as observed in our study? What about the role of FB? Shouldn't it be included in the tests, and mainly in practicing? It is few cited in literature and our study showed its importance in all the tasks proposed.

This chapter agree with the one performed by Suda et al., 2009, that found values of RMS significantly smaller results of the FL in the group of subjects with ankle instability, also a delay in response. As Santilli et al., 2005 that found in important decrease in electromyographic activity of the muscle fibularis longus in individuals with ankle instability during gait, when compared to individuals without ankle injury. On regards to TA activity, Suda et al., 2009, when investigating professional volleyball players, observed higher values of RMS in this muscle in the group with ankle instability, immediately before landing after a block. Wright et al., (2000) defend the idea that this higher activation of TA increases the risk of sprain for inversion due to an excessive supination. In the patient with sprain, it was found a higher activation of TA in the side of sprain when assessed the task with unipedal right support.

Values obtained and normalized of RMS in muscles TA, FB and FL in health volunteers might serve as a reference for studies in different lesions that involve the ankle joint. Such practice would allow a real understanding of regular and pathological patterns of muscle activation. Knowing the pattern of muscle activation involved in sprain by inversion, physiotherapy benefits with relevant information to define a protocol of treatment. A valid and conservative recommendation for clinic is the one that patients with acute and chronic history of lateral ankle sprain should be submitted to a global balance and coordination training in both limbs (Wikstrom et al., 2010).

Conclusion

It can be concluded that methodology used was sensitive in verifying differences in muscle activities. In the tasks evaluated it is highlighted an activity of fibularis brevis as an important medial-lateral stabilizer in health subjects and in the patient. However in the patient with sprain, it is observed an important activity of tibialis anterior in all tasks, in both sides that differ from low activity of fibularis longus.

References

Blackburn, J. T., Hirth, C.J. & Guskiewicz, K. M. (2003). Exercise Sandals increase lower extremity electromyographic activity during functional activities. *J Athl Train, 38*, 198–203.

Day, B. L., Steiger, M. J., Thompson, P. D. & Marsden, C. D. (1993). Effect of vision and stance width on human body motion when standing: Implications for afferent control of lateral sway. *J. Physiol*, *469*, 479-499.

Delahunt, E., Monaghan, K. & Caulfield, B. (2006). Altered neuromuscular control and ankle joint kinematics during walking in subjects with functional instability of the ankle joint. *Am J Sports Med*, *34*, 1970-1976.

Delahunt, E., McGrath, A., Doran, N. & Coughlan, G. F. (2010). Effect of Taping on Actual and Perceived Dynamic Postural Stability in Persons with Chronic Ankle Instability. *Arch Phys Med Rehab*, *91(9)*, 1383-1389.

Eechaute, C., Vaes, P., Duquet, W. & Gheluwe, B. V. (2009). Reliability and discriminative validity of sudden ankle inversion measurements in patients with chronic ankle instability. *Gait & Posture*, *30(1)*, 82-86.

Gerber, J. P., Williams, G. N., Scoville, C. R., Arciero, R. A. & Taylor, D. C. (1998). Persistent disability associated with ankle sprains: a prospective examination of an athletic population. *Foot Ankle Int*, *19(10)*, 653–660.

Hals T. M., Sitler M. R. & Mattacola C. G., (2000). Effect of a semi-rigid ankle stabilizer on performance in persons with functional ankle instability. *J Orthop Sports Phys Ther*, *30(9)*, 552–556.

Hermes H. J. & Frerik B. (2000). Development of recommendations for semg sensors and sensor placement procedures. *Journal Eletromyography kinesiology*, *10(5)*, 361-374.

Hertel J. (2000). Functional instability following lateral ankle sprain. *Sports Med*, *29(5)*, 361–371.

Horak, F. B. & Nashner, L. M. (1986). Central programming of postural movements: adaption to altered support-surface configurations. *J Neurophysiol*, *55(6)*, 1369-1381.

Johnson, M. B. & Johnson C. L. (1993). Electromyographic response of peroneal muscle in surgical and nonsurgical injured ankles during sudden inversion. *J. Orthop Sports Phys Ther*, *18*,497-501.

Kapandji, I. A. *The physiology of the joints*. Vol. 2 (Lower Limb). London: Churchill Livingstone; 2008.

Konradsen, L. & Ravn, J. B. (1991). Prolonged peroneal reaction time in ankle instability. *Int J Sports Med*, *12(3)*, 290–2.

Konradsen, L. & Magnusson, P. (2000). Increased inversion angle replication error in functional ankle instability. *Knee Surg Sports Traumatol Arthrosc*,*8(4)*, 246–251.

Konradsen, L., Olesen, S. & Hansen, H. M. (1998). Ankle sensorimotor control and eversion strength after acute ankle inversion injuries. *Am J Sports Med*, *26(1)*, 72–77.

Lofvenberg, R., Karrholm, J., Sundelin, G. & Ahlgren, O. (1995). Prolonged reaction time in patients with chronic lateral instability of the ankle. *Am J Sports Med*, *23(4)*, 414–7.

Moore, S. P., Rushmer, D. S., Windus, S. L. & Nashner, L. M. (1988) Human automatic postural responses: responses to horizontal perturbation of stance in multiple directions. *Exp Brain Res*, *73*, 648-658.

Myers, J.B., Riemann, B. L., Hwang, J. H., Fu, F. H. & Lephart, S. M. (2003). Effect of peripheral afferent alteration of the lateral ankle ligaments on dynamic stability. *Am J Sports Med*, *31(4)*, 498–506.

Osborne, M. D., Chou, L. S., Laskowski, E. R., Smith, J. & Kaufman, K. R. (2001). The effect of ankle disk training on muscle reaction time in subjects with a history of ankle sprain. *Am J Sports Med*, *29(5)*, 627–632.

Pacheco, A. M., Vaz, M. A. & Pacheco, I. (2005). Evaluation of the time for electromyographic response in volleyball athletes and non-athletes who had ankle sprain. *Rev Bras Med Esporte*, *11(6)*, 325-330.

Palmieri-Smith, R. M., Hopkins, J. T. & Brown, T. N. (2009). Peroneal activation deficits in persons with functional ankle instability. *Medicine the american journal of sports*, 982-988.

Rozendal, R. H. *Biomechanics of standing and walking*. Amsterdam: Elsevier; 1986.

Safran, M. R., Benedetti, R. S., Bartolozzi 3rd, A. R. & Mandelbaum B. R. (1999). Lateral ankle sprains: a comprehensive review: part 1: etiology, pathoanatomy,histopathogenesis, and diagnosis. *Med Sci Sports Exerc*, *31 (7)*, S429–37.

Santilli, V., Frascarelli, M. A., Paoloni, M., Frascarelli, F., Camerota, F. & Natale, F. & Santis F. (2005). Peroneus Longus Muscle Activation Pattern During Gait Cycle in Athletes Affected by Functional Ankle Instability: A Surface Electromyographic Study. The *American Journal of Sports Medicine*, *33(8)*, 1183-1187.

Shumway-Cook, A. & Woollacott, M. H. Motor control: translating research into clinical practice. Third edition. Philadelphia, Pennsylvania: Lippincott Williams & Wilkins; 2007.

Suda, E. Y., Amorim, C. F. & Sacco, I. C. N. (2009). Influence of ankle functional instability on the ankle electromyography during landing after volleyball blocking. *Journal of Electromyography and Kinesiology*, *19*, 84 – 93.

Vaes, P., Van Gheluwe, B. & Duquet, W. (2001). Control of acceleration during sudden ankle supination in people with unstable ankles. *J Orthop Sports Phys Ther*, *31(12)*, 741–52.

Wikstrom, E. A., Naik, S., Lodha N. & Cauraugh, J. H. (2010). Bilateral balance impairments after lateral ankle trauma:A systematic review and meta-analysis. *Gait & Posture*, *31(4)*, 407-414.

Wright, I. C, Neptune, R. R., Van den Bogert, A. J. Nigg, B. M. (2000). The influence of foot positioning on ankle sprains. *Journal of Biomechanics*, *33*, 513 – 519.

III) Inspiratory Muscular Activity during forward Leaning in Patients with Chronic Obstructive Pulmonary Disease (COPD)

Introduction

Forward leaning is a frequently assumed position by patients with chronic obstructive pulmonary disease (COPD) in respiratory distress in an attempt to relieve their dyspnea (O'Neill and McCarthy, 1983; Gosselink, 2003; Bott et al., 2009). It was shown that maximal inspiratory pressure (MIP) values were higher in COPD patients during forward leaning when compared to other positions, while this result was not observed in healthy adults (O'Neill and McCarthy, 1983). The superiority of this position as a generator of MIP and its association with relief of dyspnea in COPD patients is probably due at least in part to compression of abdominal contents and stretching of the diaphragm, thereby improving its length-tension relationship.

Additionally forward leaning is often associated to arm support on knees or on a surface positioned in front of them (Bott et al., 2009). Some authors have hypothesized that fixation of arms probably helps by optimizing recruitment of accessory muscles, or conversely by promoting relaxation of accessory muscle and, consequently, reducing the use of upper chest muscles (Gosselink, 2003). Although there are some studies reporting the benefits and the physiological mechanisms of forward leaning, there are still conflicting issues about the posture (Bhatt et al., 2009; Bott et al., 2009).

Based on theses findings, the aim of this chapter was to evaluate the influence of forward leaning on inspiratory muscular activity and inspired tidal volume (V_T) during the performance of breathing exercises.

Methods

Three male volunteers, aged between 60 and 70 years, one without pulmonary disease and two with moderate COPD, were evaluated. The subjects stayed seated comfortably in a chair while performing three types of breathing exercises - deep breathing and deep breathing using both flow and volume oriented incentive spirometers. The exercises were performed while assuming two thoracic positions: forward leaning and upright sitting. In all breathing exercises the subjects were instructed to execute deep inspirations up to the maximum level of volume and to sustain the inflation. During forward leaning, the volunteers stayed with their forearms placed on a stretcher in front of them and forward leaning was maintained at a 45° angle.

Inspired V_T was obtained using a ventilometer (Wright®, British Oxygen Company, London, England) and surface electromyographic activity of the following inspiratory muscles was recorded: diaphragm, external intercostals, sternocleidomastoid and scalenes. For data collection, a pair of bipolar surface electrodes was placed on the cleaned, abraded skin at each investigated muscle group from the right side of the body.

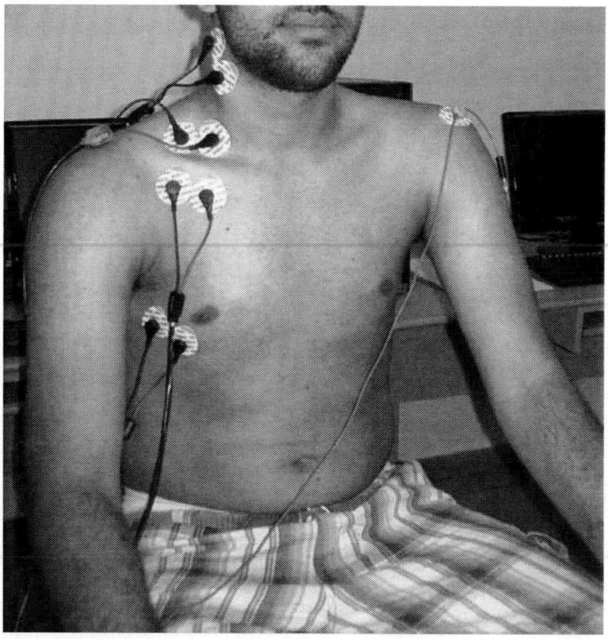

Figure 3. The placement of surface electromyographic electrodes for recording muscular activity of diaphragm, external intercostals, sternocleidomastoid and scalenes.

The electrodes to capture diaphragm activity were placed on the 7th or 8th anterior intercostal space in accordance to the best signal captured between the axillary and hemiclavicular line (de Andrade et al., 2005). To record external intercostals activity, the electrodes were placed in the 2nd or 3rd intercostal space at the midclavicular line (Chien, 2008). In the case of sternocleidomastoid, the electrodes were placed on the muscular body, at 5 cm from the mastoid process and the electrodes for recording scalenes were placed 1-2 cm above the clavicle, just behind sternocleidomastoid clavicular fibers (De Troyer et al., 1994; Hug et al., 2006). A reference electrode was placed on the coracoid process of the left scapula. Figure 3 illustrates the placement of the surface electromyographic electrodes.

For an adequate comparison of the electromyographic activities, MIP values were obtained and used to calculate the percentage of muscle activation during each breathing exercise related to the electromyographic activity recorded during MIP measurements.

Results and Discussion

Figure 4 shows inspiratory electromyographic activity obtained during the breathing exercises with the two tested thoracic positions. The graphic on the left shows inspiratory electromyographic activity of the healthy subject and the graphic on the right of the COPD volunteers. Considering all four inspiratory muscular groups, electromyographic activity does not seem to be different between the two thoracic positions, forward leaning versus upright sitting, in the COPD patients. However in the healthy subject inspiratory electromyographic activity seems to be higher during forward leaning. When evaluating individual muscle activities during the two positions, diaphragm and sternocleidomastoid electromyographic activities increased with forward leaning while external intercostals decreased and scalenes slightly increased in the healthy subject and slightly reduced in the COPDs.

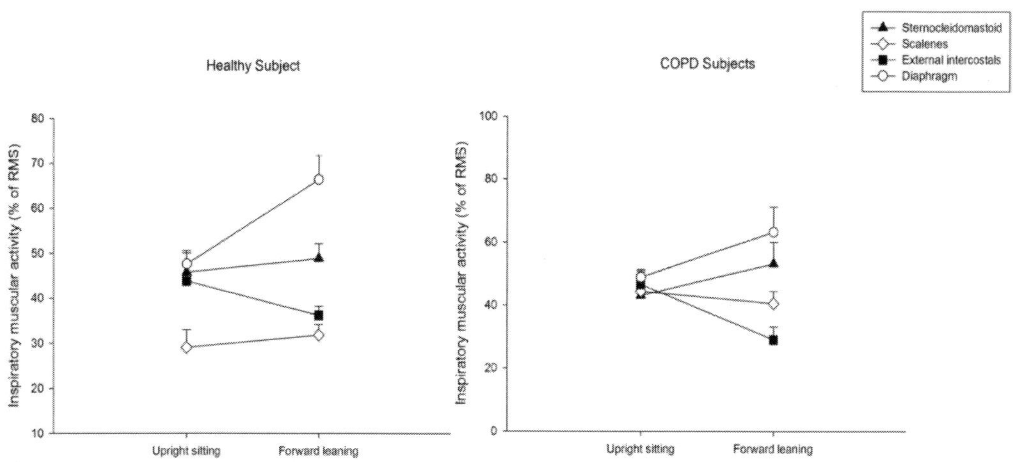

Figure 4. Inspiratory electromyographic activity obtained during the breathing exercises during the two tested thoracic positions, upright sitting versus forward leaning, in the healthy subject and in the COPD volunteers. Data are reported as means ± SE, as percentage of root mean square (RMS) values recorded during maximal inspiratory pressure measurements.

Altering thoracic position did not affect the mean inspired V_T in the healthy subject and in the COPD patients. Mean V_T was 3283 ± 104 mL and 3500 ± 100 mL in the healthy volunteer with upright sitting and forward leaning, respectively. The COPDs achieved a mean V_T of 1615 ± 339 mL with upright sitting and 1495 ± 247 mL during forward leaning.

As there is evidence that forward leaning has a positive influence on the activation pattern of inspiratory muscles in COPD patients, it was expected to occur a different response of inspiratory electromyographic activity between the healthy and the COPDs with forward leaning. This position may induce a lower work of breathing in COPD patients, i.e. forward leaning might result in a lower inspiratory electromyographic activity to mobilize a similar inspired V_T when compared with upright sitting. If it is shown that this position results a lower work of breathing, the association of forward leaning to breathing exercises during clinical attendance seems interesting due to its possible benefit – obtaining equal inspired V_T with lower energetic expenditure.

Although there is some evidence showing the benefits of forward leaning, much of this work is old and there is still some controversies requiring further investigation (Bott et al., 2009). The proposal is to continue the collects with healthy subjects and COPDs patients to better understand the effects of forward leaning on respiratory mechanics in patients with COPD.

References

Bhatt, S. P., Guleria, R., Luqman-Arafath, T. K., Gupta, A. K., Mohan, A., Nanda, S. & Stoltzfus, J. C. (2009). Effect of tripod position on objective parameters of respiratory function in stable chronic obstructive pulmonary disease. *Indian J Chest Dis Allied Sci*, *51*, 83-85.

Bott, J., Blumenthal, S., Buxton, M., Ellum, S., Falconer, C., Garrod, R., Harvey, A., Hughes, T., Lincoln, M., Mikelsons, C., Potter, C., Pryor, J., Rimington, L., Sinfield, F., Thompson, C., Vaughn, P. & White, J. (2009). Guidelines for the physiotherapy management of the adult, medical, spontaneously breathing patient. *Thorax*, *64(Suppl 1)*, i1-i51.

Chien, M. Y., Wu, Y. T. & Chang, Y. J. (2008). Assessment of diaphragm and external intercostals fatigue from surface emg using cervical magnetic stimulation. *Sensors*, *8*, 2174-2187.

de Andrade, A. D., Silva, T. N. S., Vasconcelos, H., Marcelino, M., Rodrigues-Machado, M. G.,Filho, V. C. G., Moraes, N. H., Marinho, P. E. M. & Amorim, C. F. (2005). Inspiratory muscular activation during threshold therapy in elderly healthy and patients with COPD. *J Electromyogr Kinesiol*, *15*, 631-639.

De Troyer, A., Peche, R., Yernault, J.C. & Estenne, M. (1994). Neck muscle activity in patients with severe chronic obstructive pulmonary disease. *Am J Respir Crit Care Med*, *150*, 41-47.

Gosselink, R. (2003). Controlled breathing and dyspnea in patients with chronic obstructive pulmonary disease (COPD). *J Rehabil Res Dev*, *40*, 25-33.

Hug, F., Raux, M., Prella, M., Morelot-Panzini, C., Straus, C., Similowski, T. (2006). Optimized analysis of surface electromyograms of the scalenes during quiet breathing in humans. *Respir Physiol Neurobiol*, *150*,75-81.

O'Neill, S. & McCarthy, D. S. (1983). Postural relief of dyspnoea in severe chronic airflow limitation: relationship to respiratory muscle strength. *Thorax*, *38*, 595-600.

In: Electromyography
Editor: Hiroki Takada
ISBN: 978-1- 62081-717-9

Chapter III

Bite Force, Masticatory Performance in Complete Denture Wearer: A Review

***Balendra Pratap Singh*[1], *Maneesh Kumar Singh*[2] *and Nishi Singh*[3]**
[1]Department of prosthodontics, Faculty of dental sciences,
CSM Medical University, (erstwhile King George's Medical College),
Lucknow, India
[2]Department of neurology, CSM Medical University,
(erstwhile King George's Medical College), Lucknow, India
[3]Faculty of Dental Sciences, CSM Medical University, Lucknow, India

Descriptive Abstract

Masticatory function of healthy person has been studied extensively for last decades. But, limited research has been conducted in compromised dentition. Patients with complete edentulism have a treatment of choice in the form of complete denture. Tissue supported complete denture get retention, stability and support from remaining oral tissue including facial muscles. Functional and esthetics aspect of complete denture is very much dependent upon the direction and forces generated by facial muscles. This chapter goes insight in the depth of neuromuscular control and electromyographic activity of facial muscle and how they help in stability and masticatory performance of complete denture wearer.

Introduction

Despite significant advancements in dentistry for saving teeth that previously were subject to extraction, there are literally millions of people throughout the world who have replaced their diseased teeth with dentures (Mojon P, 2003). For decades, implant therapy has been one of the notable treatment options for edentulous patients. One study highlighted the possible significant benefits for edentulous patients when using the implant technique (Zarb

GA et al, 1990). The McGill consensus statement suggested that a mandibular implant overdenture is a very powerful tool for edentulous patients (Feine JS, 2002). Many patients, unfortunately, are unable to benefit from implant treatment because of medical, psychological, or financial constraints. Therefore, conventional complete dentures remain a very important therapy for edentulous patients. Apart from improvement in speech and esthetics, most important function, challenge and requirement is mastication with complete denture.

In healthy subjects, mastication is a highly coordinated neuromuscular function that involves fast, effective movements of the jaw and continuous modulation of force. It is an alternating rhythm of isotonic and isometric contractions governed by a central pattern generator located in the brainstem (Okeson JP, 1998). Stimulation and feedback generated by sensory input from proprioceptors in the oral cavity, muscles, and joints may have an influence on the governed pattern. In older subjects, these mechanism act with marked differences. Some age-related changes, such as deterioration in the fast-and slow-twitch fibers of striated muscles, result in impaired muscle force (Grimby G, 1983). Moreover, chewing efficiency is considerably reduced when natural teeth have been replaced by complete dentures (Slagter AP, 1993). The loss of teeth and elimination of periodontal afferent flow lead to changes in the neuromuscular patterns (Veyrune JL, 2000). Edentulous persons are considered to have reduced capacity in various functions of the stomatognathic system, such as bite force, tactile thresholds, and masticatory efficiency (Slagter AP, 1992).

Edentulous State and Role of Muscles

The muscles that are intimately involved with complete denture function are skeletal muscles. Skeletal muscles are controlled by the nervous system. When a sensory nerve ending is stimulated, an afferent nerve carries the impulse to the central nervous system, where after one or more synapses, an efferent nerve will be activated, which will ultimately result in muscle contraction. This is called reflex action, as opposed to voluntary action. The reflexes occur whether we are conscious of them or not, and we do not exercise any volitional control over them; that is, we cannot start or stop them at will. The oral cavity has many sensory receptors. Many of these are associated with the periodontium. When the teeth are extracted, these receptors are lost, which means that the afferent link of some important reflexes is also lost (Zarb GA, 1982). In the ordinary sense of the term, we can voluntarily begin or stop the action of a skeletal muscle, although many skeletal muscles act when the individual is not conscious of the act. Individuals laugh, frown, scowl, and grin both consciously and subconsciously. Masticatory and nonmasticatory movements are of this same nature. A muscle can, under an individual's own volition, be activated; one muscle can be stopped and held in position, while another muscle is activated. The mandible can be in protrusion. The external pterygoid can hold the articular disk and condyle in this anteroposterior position, while the elevators and depressors can hinge the condyles on the disk. This voluntary control of skeletal muscles accounts for the stability of individuals to function in a hinge movement under their own volition (Gilman S, 1992).

Muscle is of primary interest because it performs mechanical work. Resting muscle is relatively firm but extensible. Like most tissues, it does not obey Hook's law but becomes less extensible the greater the elongation. On stimulation there is a sudden and redical change in its properties; it becomes hard, develops tension, resists stretching, and can shorten and lift a weight. The contraction occurs in the direction of the long axis of the muscle fibers. In the majority of skeletal muscles, the origins and insertions are in bone. However, many of the skeletal muscles involved in complete denture construction have a bony origin but insert into an aponeurosis, a raphe, or another muscle.

The orbicularis oris has no bony origin or insertions, and its primary function is to close the oral orifice (sphincter). When the origin and insertion of a muscle are in bone, there is a limitation to the positions and action of the muscles. When an attachment is in an aponeurosis, a raphe, or another muscle, a more flexible situation exists. With one exception, the muscles of mastication have their origins and insertions in bone, the uppermost fibers of the superior head of the external pterygoid insert into the mandibular articular capsule and thus indirectly into the anterior border of the articular disk (Zarb GA, 1982). Part of the superior head and all of the inferior head insert to the anterior surface of the mandibular neck. Knowledge of this relationship is use in making jaw relation records, particularly centric relation or centric position.

Centric Relation in Edentulous State

Centric relation is a bone-to-bone relation controlled by the attached musculature, the tissue-lined bony fossae, the ligaments, and the articular disk. It is a position that can be recorded and repeated. In the absence of a pathologic condition, individuals can return to this position under their own volition, or they can be guided such that it can be a definite point of return, provided certain other factors are understood. The functions of muscles, tendons, ligaments, and other connective tissues must be analyzed.

Muscles and tendon elasticity, extensibility, stress and fatigue, and the plastic quality of bone are some of the factors to be considered. When methods are considered for recording jaw relations, the neurological controls and their potential for distorting the record must be evaluated before any joint positions can be termed definite.

The muscle of facial expression, the muscles of the tongue, the suprahyoid muscles, the muscles of the soft palate, and the pharyngeal muscles do not have both origins and insertions in bone. These are the muscles primarily involved with determining the extent of the denture borders, the contour of the denture bases, and the positions of the teeth. The nonbony attachments of these muscles account for the various contours, borders, and positions of teeth that are seen in dentures. Impression techniques are influenced by these attachments. The muscles should not be stretched or left unsupported during an impression. The teeth, not the denture borders, support the muscles of facial expression. The available vestibular spaces should be used to their fullest extent but should not be overfilled.

Muscles Activity in Edentulous State

A muscle contraction is said to be isometric when the length of the muscle does not shorten during contraction. A muscle contraction is said to be isotonic when the muscle shortens, but the tension remains the same.

In isometric contraction, the muscle does no work, but the tension of the muscle becomes greater. Muscles contract both isomterically and isotonically in the body, with most contractions being a combination of the two. The contraction of the retractor and elevator muscles of the mandible during jaw closure is both isotonic and isometric. That is, isotonic to move the mandible and isometric to brace the jaw when the teeth contact.

When a load is placed on a muscle, the muscle elongates, and within limits, the greater the load, the greater the stretch. When the load is released, the muscle shortens almost to its original length. If the load is excessive, the muscle relaxes reflexly to keep from injuring the muscle (Yaeger JA, 1978). The property of extensibly should be considered when jaw relations are recorded under manual guidance, or when centric relation is recorded by the use of the Hickok strap.

Skeletal muscle fibers vary greatly in size from one part of the body to another. In some muscles, the fibers extend the entire length of the muscle, and usually each fiber is innervated by one neuromuscular junction located somewhere on the middle third of the fiber. A stimulus is much more effective when applied to neuromuscular junction than it is at other points of the fiber. The all-or-nothing law applies to muscle. A stimulus to a muscle fiber either causes an action potential to travel over the entire fiber or fails to stimulate it at all, except at the point of the stimulus.

The all-or-nothing law should not be interpreted to mean that if a muscle contracts, it contracts with its maximum force (Perry C, 1973). Some muscles contract very slowly and others very fast, depending on the physical and chemical characteristics of the individual muscles. The force of contraction can also vary. It can be weak or strong, depending on such variables as the presence of appropriate nutrients, or whether the fiber is already fatigued, or whether the muscle fiber is in a highly contractile state.

Moreover, the contraction of one fiber does not mean that all of the fibers in a muscle bundle are contracting. Gradation of contraction refers to the different degrees of force that can be exerted by a given muscle. A contraction of a postural muscle has slightly less gradation of contraction than that of the ocular or finger muscles. A muscle contraction is so well graded by the nervous system that almost any degree of contraction can be called forth from a muscle. The phenomenon of muscle control is one of the reasons that the reaction of the denture-supporting tissues in one individual varies from that of another because the degree of muscle contraction in a given situation can vary from person to person (Arthur O Rahn, 2002).

Another interesting property of muscle is its power to undergo physical contracture (Karkazis HC, 1998). For example, if a patient receives complete upper and lower dentures with an excessive interocclusal distance, the fibers of the elevator muscles actually shorten and re-establish new muscle lengths approximately equal to the maximum length of the lever system itself, thus re-establishing to produce optimum force of contraction. In contrast, overstretching a muscle makes its normal contraction impossible and will cause a reduction in the force of contraction.

Muscles do not act alone. When one muscle contracts, its synergist also contracts, but its antagonist must relax. When one muscle is shortened, its antagonist is stretched; this type of interaction among muscle agonist, synergist, and antagonist must be a coordinated effort to ensure efficient physiologic activity. When this purposeful muscle activity is diminished or lost, dysfunction is the result.

When muscles are at rest, a certain amount of tone usually remains. This residual degree of contraction in skeletal muscle is called muscle tone (Piancino MG, 2005). Maintenance of skeletal muscle tone depends on afferent activity from the muscle and efferent activity from the central nervous system.

The motor nerve impulses from the nervous system are coordinated with sensory information originating in the muscle spindles. The blocking of muscle spindle impulses causes loss of muscle tone, and the muscle becomes almost flaccid.

The use of drugs to inhibit the nerve impulses is sometimes advocated in the making of jaw relation records. However, the muscle relaxant drugs are not selective, and therefore their use may be quite limited in recording jaw relations.

Prolonged and strong contraction of a muscle leads to fatigue. For a fatigued muscle, the nerve, the neuromuscular junction, and even the conducting properties of the muscle membrane are normal, but the contraction becomes weaker and weaker. If a muscle becomes fatigued to an extreme extent, it is likely to become continually contracted, remaining contracted for many minutes even without an action potential as a stimulus.

If a muscle has become so fatigued that all the energy giving compounds have been degraded, relaxation cannot be provided, and the muscle assumes a prolonged contracted state.

When the fatigue is over, the muscle gradually relaxes. If an individual's mandible is protruded and allowed to remain until fatigue occurs, the antagonist action of the retractor and elevator muscles will be weakened.

It wound be possible to retrude and elevate the mandible to centric position against very little or no opposing action from the lateral pterygoid. However, care must be exercised not to keep the mandible in protrusion until extreme fatigue exists. This could defeat the purpose, at least for many minutes, as the lateral pterygoid could become continually contracted.

Parallelogram of Muscular Forces in Prosthesis Wearer

From the standpoint of the prosthodontics, the skull presents some interesting facts that need to be taken into consideration. The factor of muscle pull in relation to the direction and strength of each individual muscle used in positioning the mandible after the loss of teeth is an important consideration.

The parallelogram of forces can be studied only in relation to the entire skull. The direction of these forces has much to do with the seating or unseating dentures. The occlusal vertical dimension affects this direction of forces, a fact that makes the positioning of the mandible after the loss of teeth so important.

One can understand the relation of the ridges by studying the teeth in the natural occlusion or observe the inclination of the roots and the alveolar process.

A study of the skull as a whole in relation to the attaching muscles and their consequent pull should reveal the hazard of placing the mandible anterior to its centric position. There is only one true centric relation, and that coincides with the center of muscle pull when the mandible is in its most retruded position in relation to the skull (Judson C Hickey, 1983).

Different Treatment Modalities and Muscles Activity

1. Tissue Supported Complete Denture

A. Mastication with Complete Denture

Observation of the effect of tooth loss in elderly individuals shows that the presence of natural teeth allows a better masticatory performance compared to the use removable complete dentures with regards to masticatory efficiency, masticatory time, selection of more consistent foods (Wayler AH, 1983) and electromyographic activity (Kapur KK, 1984). Within this context, edentulous individuals wearing removable completer dentures exhibit reduced muscular activity at the working side, which is poorly adapted to the food texture, as well as decreased electromyographic activity, especially of the masseter muscle, when compared to dentate individuals (Veyrune JL, 2000). The stability of complete dentures also influences the masticatory performance of individuals, as damages to this aspect would result in less regularity and uniformity of mastication cycles (Karkazis, HC, 1998). Moreover, use of prostheses damages the sensitivity, oral stereognosis and taste and may also influence the feeding, swallowing and nutritional status of elderly individuals (Ship JA, 1996).

Regarding the adaptation to new dentures, edentulous elderly individuals wearing removable complete dentures for several years exhibit temporary reduction in activity of the masseter muscle at the working side after placement of new dentures, while the activity of the anterior temporalis muscle remains reduced (Piancino MG, 2005).

B. Masticatory Muscles Activity in Complete Denture Rehabilitated Subjects

A study by Iva Z. Alajbeg et al (Alajbeg IZ, 2005) have shown that maximal elevator muscle activity levels in intercuspal position were higher in dentate subjects than in edentulous subjects, while during maximal wide opening, depressor muscle activity levels were similar in dentulous and edentulous subjects. Considering elevator muscle activity during the maximal clenching trial, their results were in agreement with those of other authors, (Karkazis HC, 1998; Kawamura U, 1967) who had reported that denture wearers were unable to produce levels of muscle activity at maximal voluntary contraction comparable to those in subjects with natural teeth. Miralles et al (Kawamura U, 1964) showed that low muscle activity in patients with complete dentures might be a consequence of a change in the influence of peripheral or central neural mechanisms, since in edentulous patients the periodontal receptors are missing, and mucosal mechanoreceptors play the main role in replacing them. Change in the input from peripheral receptors and their influence on trigeminal motor neuron pools could be expected with the loss of natural teeth. In the study of Proeschel and Raum, (Proeschel PA, 2003) included healthy dentate subjects; the digastrics muscles produced the highest activity during a mandible-balancing trial, while depressor activation during chewing exceeded depressor activation during clenching. No reports, however, have been devoted to the study of these factors in denture wearers.

Although numerous studies have described normal masticatory performance in young adults and children, (Julien KC, 1996; Saifuddin M, 2001) little comparative information has been shown regarding the differences in mastication between dentate and edentulous subjects of similar age. Impairments induced by replacement of natural teeth by complete dentures have been described with regard to bite force; tongue motor skill, and chewing efficiency measured by the quality of comminution (Slagter AP, 1993; Slagter AP, 1992; Ingervall B, 1980). Subject satisfaction has been examined in various surveys in terms of subjective criteria, such as chewing ability, chewing comfort, stability, and speech, (Feine JS, 1994; Garrett NR, 1996; Gunne HS, 1985) but the results could not completely clarify whether the functional capacity of edentulous patients' masticatory system is reduced in comparison to dentate subjects. Considering muscle activity during chewing, as presented in the study of Alajbeg (2005), it is obvious that higher values of myoelectrical signals (in microvolt) were found in dentate subjects than in complete denture wearers during five sequences of mastication. However, the amounts of muscle activity in proportion to maximal activity were higher in edentulous subjects when compared to age-matched dentate subjects. This indicates that the elevator and depressor muscles in the edentulous subjects changes their pattern, compared to the dentulous subjects, to perform optimal mastication with the reduced absolute muscle activity as a result of denture insertion and protective reflex mechanisms of neuromuscular control. Few more studies have shown that (Berretin-Felix G, 2008; Miralles R, 1989) edentulous subjects had to use a significantly higher potential of muscle activity than dentate subjects during mastication. This finding add to the knowledge of mastication the fact that edentulous subjects, while chewing with dentures, involve more masticatory muscle fibers than dentate subjects, and gradually decrease muscle contractions, probably because of fatigue. This showed that complete denture wearers were functionally inferior to subjects with natural dentition, and therefore had to change their muscle activity patterns which led to an inability to increase muscle activity at the end of chewing task. Reduced muscle activity and a difference in the chewing pattern should be explained to a patient prior to prosthodontics rehabilitation with complete dentures, so that they can adjust their expectations.

2. Tooth and Implant Supported Overdenture

A. Physiology of Tooth and Implant Supported Prosthesis

The contact between maxillary and mandibular teeth in different functions is monitored primarily by mechanoreceptors in the periodontal ligament (PDL). Stimulation of the afferent sensory impulses relays information to synapses and the central nervous system, (Hassanali J, 1997) resulting in an efferent response and the initiation of muscular activity (Mericske-Stern R, 1993). When a patient loses one or more teeth, there is loss of function, impaired esthetics, and loss of the PDL and its mechanoreceptors. A prosthetic replacement may require a re-adaptation of the central and periphery neuromuscular complex. Osseointegrated implants provide new treatment options for patients (Zarb GA, 1990 part I,II,III; Branemark PI, 1985; Smith DE, 1989). Tissue-implant integration is achieved by direct contact of bone with the implant surface, establishing implant ankylosis. This direct bone-implant contact omits the PDL and its mechanoreceptors and may influence the pattern of masticatory function.

Patients treated with implant-supported prostheses may adapt to the new neuromuscular feedback environment, thus establishing a unique coordination pattern of masticatory muscles. Gartner et al (2000) investigated the long-term effect of osseointegration implant therapy on functional outcome and stated that patients with implant-supported prostheses appeared to be well adapted to perform habitual masticatory functions. However, during a nonhabitual function such as maximal occluding force, Gartner et al revealed a less coordinated masticatory muscle activity in the implant patients. In a study of adaptation to the new prostheses, Mushimoto et al (1988) reported that well-coordinated masticatory muscle activities were reestablished in patients with a tissue-supported prosthesis one month after prosthesis insertion. In a study by Gartner et al (2000), volunteers with implant had used the final prosthesis for at least six months at the time of examination. Electromyographic analysis of masticatory muscles during habitual chewing indicated that the muscle activity of the implant group was generally smaller than that of the control group. Otherwise, the descriptive differences between implant and dentulous subjects' masticatory muscle coordination patterns were not statistically significant. Implant patients in this study appeared well-adapted to the implant-supported prostheses for habitual functions. These studies may suggest that during adaptation to the implant supported prosthesis, remote proprioceptive receptors might be activated through transmission of vibrations through the jawbone, (Jacobs R, 1995) for which the lost PDL-derived proprioceptive mechanism for habitual chewing coordination could be compensated (Jacobs R, 1994). However, it is tempting to speculate that the implant patients may acquire new muscle coordination through a different neuromuscular network, which might be particularly emphasized during a nonhabitual activity.

B. Masticatory Performance with Tooth and Implant Supported Prosthesis

The type of dental treatment performed in adults and elderly individuals also influences the masticatory efficiency, which is greater in individuals rehabilitated with tooth supported and implant-supported dentures compared to removable complete dentures. It should be highlighted that individuals wearing tooth-supported dentures exhibit greater electromyographic activity of the anterior temporalis muscle during masticatory function, both in the amplitude and value of integrated activity, compared to individuals wearing removable complete and implant-supported dentures in the mandibular arch (Chen L, 2002). Thus, the use of implant-supported prostheses leads to improved masticatory function characterized by an increase in electromyographic activity and reduced masticatory cycle time (Bakke M, 2002) although neuromuscular coordination is lower compared to individuals with natural teeth (Ferrario VF, 2004).

A study by Giédre Berretin-Felix et al (2008) evaluated the muscular activity involved in processes of mastication on rubber and swallowing of foods of different textures in elderly individuals using electromyography to compare their performance before and after placement of implant-supported prostheses in the mandibular arch. The results showed statistically significant reduction in bioelectric activity after implant supported oral rehabilitation in the masseter muscles for swallowing of both paste and liquid foods. Differences were more marked when preoperative values were compared to 6 and 18 months post treatment. Similar performance was observed for the submental muscles, yet without statistically significant difference. The orbicularis oris muscle presented increased activity at all post-implant periods for mastication on rubber, yet without statistically significant difference in results between periods. The reduction of muscular activity after implant supported oral rehabilitation observed in this study is different from the findings of other investigations that reported increased masticatory activity after implant placement (Chen L, 2002; Bakke M, 2002). Karkazis HC (2002) also concluded that rehabilitation with implant retained mandibular dentures may result in more regular chewing patterns with higher electrical activity of the masseter muscles, thus providing improved chewing function and comfort. However, Chen et al (2002) investigated adults and elderly and observed lower amplitude results for the masseter muscle in the group treated with implant supported dentures, in agreement with the findings of the present study.

Conversely, Haraldson et al (1979) Haraldson and Inger-Vall (1979) verified that electromyographic activity related to the masticatory muscles and the superior orbicularis oris muscle in adult women wearing implant-supported prostheses was similar to those with natural teeth at the same age range. The presence of numerically lower values for the submental muscles after implant-supported oral rehabilitation seems to be associated to physiological adjustments expected during the aging process, since studies conducted on dentate individuals found reduction in electromyographic amplitude with age (Vaiman M, 2004; Vaiman M, 2004).

Moreover, the greater activity of masseter and suprahyoid muscles preoperatively might be explained by the recruitment of a larger number of motor units to retain mandibular removable dentures.

According to Veyrune and Mioche (2000) tooth loss and use of complete dentures affects the motor and sensorial aspects involved in the masticatory process. Information received centrally is not sufficiently accurate to allow adaptation of mastication patterns to the food texture in denture wearers. It should be highlighted that the loss of teeth and consequently of periodontal receptors impairs the sensorial biofeedback (Kawamura U, 1964) mainly due to information from the mechanoreceptors and muscle spindles (Kawamura U, 1967). Adaptation of the stomatognathic system to the anatomic-physiological conditions of individuals is certainly responsible for the partial release of mandibular elevator muscles after achievement of stabilization by placement of implant supported dentures, inducing a decrease in muscular activity in the postoperative period.

The opposite occurred in the case of the orbicularis oris muscle, where the probable loss of coordination or the need to adjust the maxillary removable prosthesis to the mandibular fixed prosthesis could have caused increased muscle activity in an attempt to hold the maxillary prosthesis in place.

Thus, the results indicate that use of implant-supported fixed dentures leads to physiological adaptations to the oral condition and aging process. One study on improvement and long-term stability of neuromuscular adaptation in implant-supported overdenture showed that treatment with two interforaminal implants provides evidence of neuromuscular adaptation towards values of healthy dentate.

Thus, the known benefits of implant placement such as tissue perseverance and improved function are complemented by improved neuromuscular adaptation.

Conclusion

It was concluded that rehabilitation with implant retained denture may result in more regular chewing patterns with higher electrical activity of the masseter muscles, thus providing improved chewing function and comfort.

References

Alajbeg, I. Z., Valentic-Peruzovic, M., Alajbeg, I., Illes, D., & Celebic, A. (2005). The influence of dental status on masticatory muscle activity in elderly patients. *Int J Prosthodont,18,*333-338.

Arthur O. R., & Charles M. H. Jr (2002). *Textbook of complete denture: Anatomy and Physiology* (Fifth edition). Noida, India: Private Limited.

Bakke, M., Holm, B., & Gotfredsen, K. (2002). Masticatory function and patient satisfaction with implant-supported mandibular overdentures: a prospective 5-year study. *Int J Prosthodont, 15,* 575-581.

Berretin-Felix, G., Nary Filho, H., Padovani, C. R., Trindade JR., A. S., & Machado W. M. (2008). Electromyographic evaluation of mastication and swallowing in elderly individuals with mandibular fixed implant-supported prostheses. *J Appl Oral Sci, 16,* 116-121.

Brånemark, P. I., Zarb, G. A., & Albrektsson, T. (1985). *Tissue-integrated prosthesis: Osseointegration in clinical dentistry.* Chicago, IL: Quintessence Publishing.

Chen, L., Xie, Q., Feng, H., Lin, Y., & Li, J. (2002). The masticatory efficiency of mandibular implant-supported overdentures as compared with tooth-supported overdentures and complete dentures. *J Oral Implantol, 28,* 238-243.

Feine, J. S., Carlsson, G. E., Awad, M. A. Chehade, A., Duncan, W. J., Gizani, S., Head, T., Heydecke, G., Lund, J. P., MacEntee, M., Mericske-Stern, R., Mojon, P., Morais, J. A., Naert, I., Payne, A. G., Penrod, J., Stoker, G. T., Tawse-Smith, A., Taylor, T. D., Thomason, J. M., Thomson, W. M., & Wismeijer, D. (2002). The McGill consensus statement on overdentures. Montreal, Quebec, Canada. May 24-25, 2002. *Int J Prosthodont, 15 (4),* 413-414.

Feine, J. S., Maskawi, K., de Grandmont, P., Donohue, W. B., Tanguay, R., & Lund, J. P. (1994). Within-subject comparisons of implant-supported mandibular prostheses: evaluation of masticatory function. *J Dent Res, 73,* 1646-1656.

Ferrario, V. F., Tartaglia G. M., Maglione, M., Simion, M., & Sforza, C. (2004). Neuromuscular coordination of masticator muscles in subjects with two types of implant-supported prostheses. *Clin Oral Implant Res, 15,* 219-225.

Garrett, N. R., Perez, P., Elbert, C., & Kapur, K. K. (1996). Effects of improvements of poorly fitting dentures and new dentures on masseter activity during chewing. *J Prosthet Dent, 76,* 394-402.

Gartner, J. L., Mushimoto, K., Weber, H. P., & Nishimura, I. (2000). Effect of osseointegrated implants on the coordination of masticatory muscles: a pilot study. *J Prosthet Dent, 84,* 185-193.

Gilman, S. & Newman, S. W. (1992). *Manter and Gatz's Essentials of clinical neuroanatomy and neurophysiology* (8th edition). Philadelphia, PA: F.A. Davis Company.

Grimby, G. & Saltin, B. (1983). The ageing muscle. *Clin Physiol, 3,* 209-218.

Gunne, H. S. & Wall, A. K. (1985). The effect of new complete dentures on mastication and dietary intake. *Acta Odontol Scand, 43,* 257-268.

Haraldson, T., Carlsson, G. E., & Ingervall, B. (1979). Functional state, bite force and postural muscle activity in patients with osseointegrated oral implant bridges. *Acta Odontol Scand, 37,* 195-206.

Haraldson, T. & Ingervall, B. (1979). Muscle function during chewing and swallowing in patients with osseointegrated oral implant bridges: An electromyographic study. *Acta Odontol Scand*, *37*, 207-216.

Hassanali, J. (1997). Quantitative and somatotopic mapping of neurones in the trigeminal mesencephalic nucleus and ganglion innervating teeth in monkey and baboon. *Arch Oral Biol*, *42*, 673-682.

Ingervall, B. & Hedegard, B._(1980). An electromyographic study of masticatory and lip muscle function in patients with complete dentures. *J Prosthet Dent*, *43*, 266-271.

Jacobs, R. & van Steenberghe, D. (1994). Role of periodontal ligament receptors in the tactile function of teeth: a review. *J Periodontal Res*, *29*, 153-167.

Jacobs, R. & van Steenberghe, D. (1995). Qualitative evaluation of the masseteric poststimulus EMG complex following mechanical or acoustic stimulation of osseointegrated oral implants. *Int J Oral Maxillofac Implants*, *10*, 175-182.

Hickey, J. C., Zarb, G. A., & Bolender, C. L. (1990). *Biological considerations of jaw relations and jaw movements: Prosthodontic treatment for edentulous patients* (ninth edition). Delhi, India: B C Decker.

Julien, K. C., Buschang, P. H., Throckmorton, G. S., & Dechow, P. C. (1996). Normal masticatory performance in young adults and children. *Arch Oral Biol*, *41*, 69-75.

Kapur, K. K. & Garrett, N. R. (1984). Studies of biologic parameters for denture design. Part II: comparison of masseter muscle activity, masticatory performance, and salivatory secretion rates between denture and natural dentition groups. *J Prosthet Dent*, *52*, 408-413.

Karkazis, H. C. (2002). EMG activity of the masseter muscle in implant supported overdenture wearers during chewing of hard and soft food. *J Oral Rehabil*, *29*, 986-991.

Karkazis, H. C. & Kossioni, A. E. (1998). Surface EMG activity of the masseter muscle in denture wearers during chewing of hard and soft food. *J Oral Rehabil*, *25*, 8-14.

Kawamura, U. (1967). Neurophysiology background of occlusion. *Periodontics*, *5*, 175-183.

Kawamura, U. & Majima, T. (1964). Temporomandibular-joint's sensory mechanisms controlling activities of the jaw muscles. *J Dent Res*, *43*, 150.

Mericske-Stern, R., Hofmann, J., Wedig, A. & Geering, A. H. (1993). In vivo measurements of maximal occlusal force and minimal pressure threshold on overdentures supported by implants or natural roots: a comparative study, part I. *Int J Oral Maxillofac Implants*, *8*, 641-649.

Miralles, R., Berger, B., Ide, W., Manns, A., Bull, R. & Carvajal, A. (1989). Comparative electromyographic study of elevator muscles in patients with complete dentures and natural dentition. *J Oral Rehabil*, *16*, 249-255.

Mojon, P. (2003). The world without teeth: Demographic trends. In: J. S. Feine, & G. E. Carlsson (Eds.), *Implant Overdentures: The standard of care for edentulous patients* (edition 2, pp. 3-14). Chicago, IL: Quintessence.

Mushimoto, E., Kawani, A., Ohi, H., Tatsuta, T., & Mitani, H. (1988). Functional significance of pressure sensation conveyed by removable partial dentures. *Int J Prosthodont*, *1*, 41-45.

Okeson, J. P. (1998). *Management of Temporomandibular Disorders and Occlusion* (Fifth edition). St Louis, MO: Mosby.

Perry, C. (1973). Neuromuscular control of mandibular movements. *J Prosthet Dent*, *30*, 714-720.

Piancino, M. G., Farina, D., Talpone, F., Castroflorio, T., Gassino, G., Margarino, V., & Bracco, P. (2005). Surface EMG of jaw-elevator muscles and chewing pattern in complete denture wearers. *J Oral Rehabil*, *32*, 863-870.

Porter, M. R. (1970). The attachment of lateral pterygoid muscle to meniscus. *J Prosthet Dent*, *24*, 555-562.

Proeschel, P. A. & Raum, J. (2003). Task-dependence of jaw elevator and depressor co-activation. *J Dent Res*, *82*, 617-620.

Saifuddin, M., Miyamoto, K., Ueda, H. M., Shikata, N., & Tanne, K. (2001). A quantitative electromyographic analysis of masticatory muscle activity in usual daily life. *Oral Dis*, *7*, 94-100.

Ship, J. A., Duffy, V., Jones, J. A., & Langmore, S. (1996). Geriatric oral health and its impact on eating. *J Am Geriatr Soc*, *44*, 456-464.

Slagter, A. P., Bosman, F., van der Glas, H. W., & van der Bilt, A. (1993). Human jaw-elevator muscle activity and food comminution in the dentate and edentulous state. *Arch Oral Biol*, *38*, 195-205.

Slagter, A. P., Olthoff, L. W., Bosman, F., & Steen, W. H. (1992). Masticatory ability, denture quality, and oral conditions in edentulous subjects. *J Prosthet Dent*, *68*, 299-307.

Smith, D. E., & Zarb, G. A. (1989). Criteria for success of osseointegrated endosseous implants. *J Prosthet Dent*, *62*, 567-572.

Vaiman, M., Eviatar, E., & Segal, S. (2004). Surface electromyographic studies of swallowing in normal subjects: a review of 440 adults. Report 1. Quantitative data: timing measures. *Otolaryngol Head Neck Surg*, *131*, 548-555.

Vaiman, M., Eviatar, E., & Segal, S. (2004). Surface electromyographic studies of swallowing in normal subjects: a review of 440 adults. Report 2. Quantitative data: amplitude measures. *Otolaryngol Head Neck Surg*, *131*, 773-780.

Veyrune, J. L. & Mioche, L. (2000). Complete denture wearers: electromyography of mastication and texture perception whilst eating meat. *Eur J Oral Sci*, *108*, 83-92.

Wayler, A.H. & Chauncey, H. H. (1983). Impact of complete dentures and impaired natural dentition on masticatory performance and food choice in healthy aging men. *J Prosthet Dent*, *49*, 427-433.

Yaeger, J. A. (1978). Mandibular path in the grinding phase of mastication- a review. *J Prosthet Dent*, *39*, 569-573.

Zarb, G. A. (1982). Oral motor patterns and their relation to oral prostheses. *J Prosthet Dent*, *47*, 472-478.

Zarb, G. A. & Schmitt, A. (1990). The longitudinal clinical effectiveness of osseointegrated dental implants: the toronto study. Part 1: Surgical result. *J Prosthet Dent*, *63*, 451-457.

Zarb, G. A. & Schmitt, A. (1990). The longitudinal clinical effectiveness of osseointegrated dental implants: The Toronto study. Part II: The prosthetic results. *J Prosthet Dent*, *64*, 53-61.

Zarb, G. A. & Schmitt, A. (1990). The longitudinal clinical effectiveness of osseointegrated dental implants: The Toronto study. Part III: Problems and complications encountered. *J Prosthet Dent*, *64*, 185-194.

Reviewed by:

1. Dr Atul Bhatnagar
   Associate professor
   Faculty of dentistry
   Institute of medical sciences
   Banaras Hindu University
   Varanasi
   Email: atuldent@hotmail.com
2. Dr Saranjit singh bhasin
   Professor
   Department of prosthodontics
   Faculty of dentistry
   Jamia Millia Islamia
   New delhi 110025
   Email: drsmyle@yahoo.com

In: Electromyography
Editor: Hiroki Takada

ISBN: 978-1- 62081-717-9

Chapter IV

Sensor Output Signal Evaluation System for Biofeedback Training and Its Apprication

***Tomoki Shiozawa*[1*], *Hiroki Takada*[2], *Yasuyuki Matsuura*[3] and *Masaru Miyao*[4]**

[1] Aoyama Gakuin University, Shibuya, Shibuya-ku, Tokyo, Japan
[2] Graduate School of Engineering, University of Fukui, Fukui, Japan
[3] Headquarters for Innovative Society-Academic Cooperation, University of Fukui, Fukui, Japan
[4] Graduate School of Information Science, Nagoya University, Chikusa-ku, Nagoya, Japan

Abstract

To improve the self-control ability of a specific muscle, a technique called biofeedback training can be used, which presents the subject with electromyography (EMG) waveforms that are generated either by the subject or mathematical analyses. The waveforms are usually presented to subjects visually or aurally. This section outlines the methodologies of EMG and the problems encountered in these methodologies, and introduces biofeedback training (BFT) using surface EMG. In addition, a "sensor output evaluation system," which evaluates BFT by quantifying and analyzing sEMG and its integrated waveform, is explained and the future of this technology is discussed.

Introduction

Several electromyographic methods are currently used, but needle electromyography (nEMG) and surface electromyography (sEMG) are most often applied. To physiologically

* shiozawa@busi.aoyama.ac.jp.

evaluate electromyographic wave patterns for the detection of abnormalities, wave patterns obtained with nEMG or sEMG have been macroscopically examined, and subjectively judged by physicians.

A) nEMG findings are used to classify a disorder as neurogenic or myogenic. In the case where a disorder is both neurogenic and myogenic, nEMG findings provide important information about whether it the disorder is acute, sub acute, or chronic (Kimura, 1989). However, a needle electrode probe is used, which is percutaneously inserted into muscular tissue.
B) sEMG findings are used for various evaluations, such as the classification of trembling for the diagnosis of involuntary motion, the diagnosis or differential diagnosis of dystonia and spasm, and the identification of involuntary constrictor muscles (Kizuka et al., 2006).
C) sEMG is also used for the determination of the electric potential through a nerve conduction examination (this procedure is called evoked EMG). In evoked EMG, the electrostimulation of peripheral nerves is performed percutaneously (Kimura, 1989). Nerve conduction study (often called a nerve conduction examination) (Figure 1) can reveal the following findings;

1) decay of nerve conduction velocity (demyelination)
2) attenuated amplitude of evoked electromyogram (axonal motor neuropathy)
3) attenuated amplitude of sensory nerve action potential (axonal sensory neuropathy)
4) temporal dispersion of electromyogram (existence of demyelinating disorder)
5) attenuation (myasthenia gravis) or amplification (Lambert-Eaton myasthenic syndrome) of evoked potential due to repetitive stimulation
6) conduction block (demyelination)
7) delay of central motor conduction time (motor conduction disturbance of central nervous system)

The examination methods described, except for method B), are invasive and cause severe pain in patients. “Smoothing” and “integration” refer to two ways of quantifying EMG energy over time. Smoothing refers to continuously averaging out the peaks and valleys of a changing electrical signal, and integration refers to measuring the area under a curve over a period of time. These methods are used to examine the relative degree of muscular contraction, and are also employed to provide parameters for the evaluation of muscular training conditions (Aukee, 2002). However, the results obtained are affected by the location of the measuring electrodes and the shape and size of the probes. This means that although EMG findings are macroscopically and subjectively evaluated, as described above, no algorithm for the quantification of the degree of muscular abnormalities or recovery has been established. In this study, we applied the measurement parameters that have been developed for evaluating the average rectified sEMG (ARS) data obtained from perineal muscles during biofeedback training (BFT) for the treatment of dysuria (Tries & Eisman, 1995) and evaluated the effects of this training (Shiozawa et al., 2007). We discuss the results in a later section of this chapter. Kegel (1948; 1951) was the first to use BFT for the treatment of urinary incontinence (UI), and it was observed that if the pelvic floor muscles were hypotonic, bladder suspension surgery was less effective for treating stress-related incontinence. In order to improve the contractibility of the pubococcygeus portion of the levator ani muscle, Kegel invented the pressure perineometer (Kegel, 1948; Kegel, 1951).

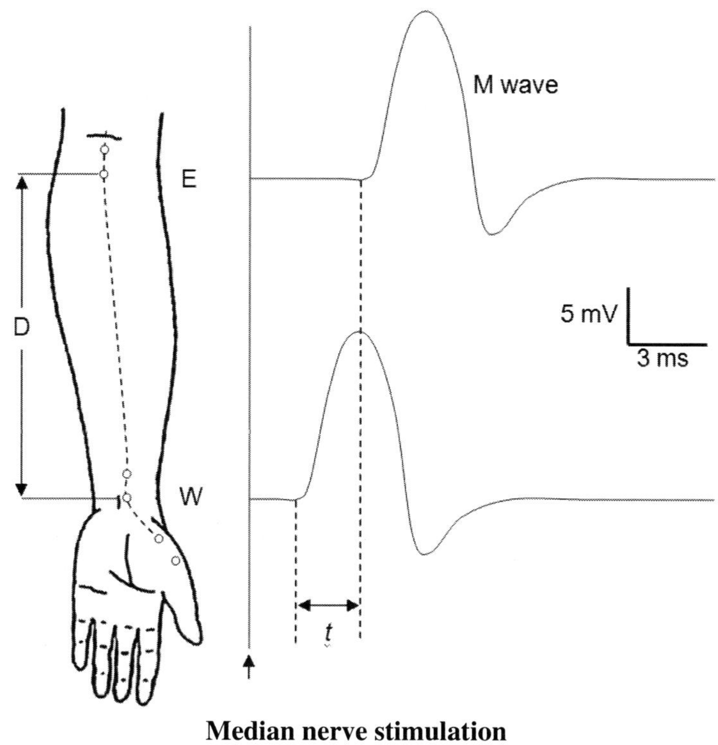

Figure 1. Nerve conduction study of the median nerve. M waves obtained from the abductor pollicis brevis muscle by stimulating the wrist and elbow joints. Motor conduction velocity = D/*t*.

A biofeedback instrument has three tasks to perform (Peek et al., 1995): first, to monitor (in some way) a physiological process of interest, second, to measure (objectify) what is monitored, and third, to present what is monitored or measured as meaningful information. There are many researchers and practitioners that can be cited as forerunners of biofeedback.

Edmund Jacobsen commenced research at Harvard in 1908, and throughout the 1920s and 1930s worked to develop progressive muscle relaxation as an effective behavioral technique for the alleviation of neurotic tensions and many functional medical disorders (Jacobsen, 1938). He used crude electromyographic equipment to monitor the levels of muscle tension in his patients during the course of treatment. The classification of and historical perspectives on biofeedback applications can be found in reports by Gaarder and Montgomery (1981), Gatchel and Price (1979), and Basmajian (1989)).

Recently, the rapid atrophy of the muscles used for bending at the hip joint during walking (i.e., the flexor muscles around the hip joint) with age has drawn attention. The flexor muscles around the hip joint consist of the femoral rectus and abdominal muscles. It has been indicated that a lack of strength in these muscles is responsible for many of the falls suffered by the elderly. In this study, we examined the ARS of the femoral rectus muscles performed during the BFT of the dominant leg using the measurement parameters mentioned above, and evaluated changes in these parameters with age.

Sensor output Signal Evaluation System

The sensor output signal evaluation (SOSE) system was developed in 2006 (Shiozawa et al., 2006a). The SOSE system can evaluate the exponential curve-fitting in BFT.

Participants

The subjects consisted of 31 healthy adults aged 20-73 years (mean, 44.3±19.9 years). All of the subjects were Japanese and lived in Nagoya and its environs. The following were the exclusion criteria for the subjects: subjects working in a night shift, subjects with a dependence on alcohol, subjects who consumed alcohol and caffeine-containing beverages after waking up and within two hours of eating a meal, subjects who may have had a previous history of bone, joint, or nerve problems, and special strength training exercises were not usually done. The subjects were not prescribed drugs for any disease.

Design

The subject sat back on a four-legged stool, and electromyographic electrodes were applied at an interval of several centimeters to the center of the femoral rectus muscles in the dominant left or right leg (Figure 2). The subjects were instructed to kick a fixed belt by moving the bottom of the lower leg forward (kicking motion).

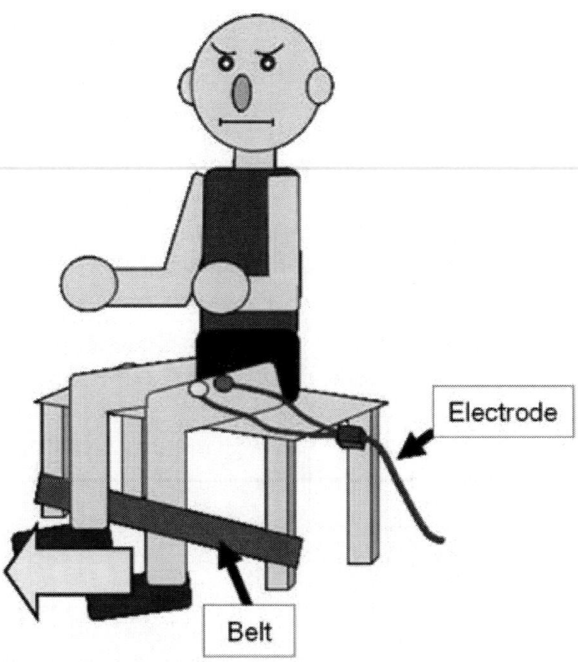

Figure 2. Biofeedback training of femoral rectus mescles.

Biofeedback Training

Temporal data were obtained using sEMG, and they are expressed here as $\{y(t)\}$. Generally, sEMG data are recorded by a computer at 2 kHz. Here, the integral calculation was performed every 0.1 s using the following equation:

$$x(t) = \sum_{k=0}^{199} \left| y(t + 0.0005k) \right| \tag{1}$$

and the ARS $\{x(t)\}$ was calculated in real time and outputted. The subject was told to observe the outputted wave patterns and the rectangular waves $f(t)$ of a 10-s cycle superimposed on the same display (Figure 3), and then perform intermittent continuous contractions of the femoral rectus muscles corresponding to the patterns (BFT). The subjects performed BFT for 2 min. We ensured that the body sway was not affected by environmental conditions; using an air conditioner, we adjusted the *temperature* to 25 °C in the exercise room, which was large, quiet, and *bright*. All subjects were tested from 10 am to 5 pm in an exercise *room*. All subjects gave consent in writing after a sufficient explanation of this study.

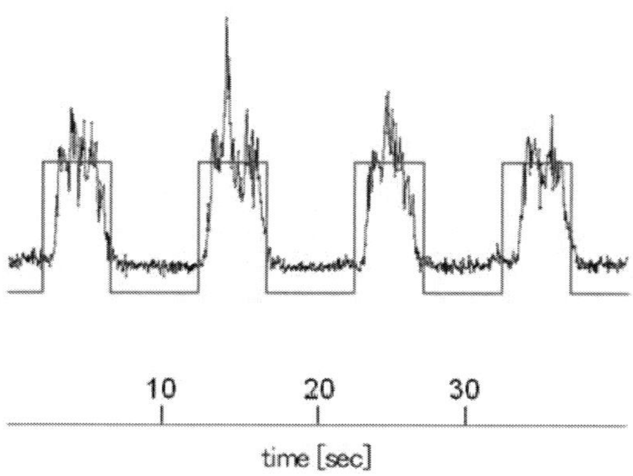

Figure 3. Biofeedback training instruction signal. The BFT instruction signal produced by superimposing the ARS on the target instruction signal.

Materials

A special electromyographic transformation box (AP-U027, TEAC Co.) was connected to a commercially available portable and versatile amplifier and recorder (Polymate AP1532, TEAC Co.), and electromyographic electrodes (bipolar) with preamplifiers were used.

Procedure

First, the electromyographic wave patterns obtained over 5 seconds at the maximum effort of the kicking motion (maximum voluntary contraction (MVC) (Carlo and Deluca,

1997) were integrated in real time using a computer, and the ARS data on the display were shown to the subject. Next, the threshold line at 75% of the mean ARS (mV) during the muscular contraction period was shown to the subject, who was requested to perform muscular training aiming at the threshold line for 1 min 20 s. In other words, BFT was performed at 75% of the MVC. During BFT, data were recorded in a notebook computer (AP Monitor, NoruPro) at a sampling rate of 2 kHz. The low frequency cut-off filters were used at 16 Hz, and an alternating current-eliminating filter was also used.

Algorithm in the SOSE System

The initial 20 s of the sEMG data recorded over a total of 1 min 20 s were excluded, because the subjects may have required this time to adjust to the training. The sEMG data of the 6-cycle rectangular waves that occurred over the remaining minutes of training (target value) and the ARS were analyzed in accordance with the Double-Wayland algorithm (Takada et al., 2006a) and our own mathematical algorithms of the sensor output signal evaluation system. Figure 4 shows a revision of the flow chart in Shiozawa et al. (2006). Taking a mean of the ARS (MARS) as a threshold H for determining continuous muscular contractions, the time sequences above the threshold H were regarded as continuous muscular contractions. Based on whether differences such as $x(t) - x(t - 0.1)$ and $(x(t + 0.1) - x(t))(x(t) - x(t - 0.1))$ were positive or negative, a maximal series for the continuous muscular contractions was extracted as shown in Figure 5.

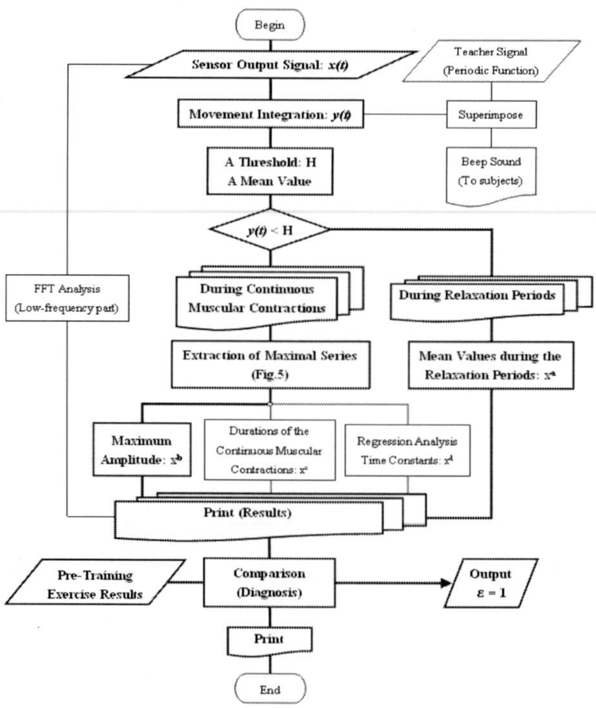

Figure 4. A part of the flow chart of our mathematical algorithm of the sensor output signal evaluation (SOSE) system. The SOSE system counts the number of muscular contraction periods and determines whether the muscles work normally.

a) The value of the MARS during the muscular relaxation period (xa) and the measurement parameters in the other terms (Shiozawa et al., 2006b; Shiozawa et al., 2006c; Takada et al., 2006b) indicating the shape of the ARS were determined every cycle, and the ARS values obtained from the femoral rectus muscles were evaluated.

(b) Maximum amplitude (xb): This maximum value was examined and recorded.

(c) Duration of continuous muscular contraction (x^c). The duration between the first and last maximal values in a cycle exceeding the MARS sEMG was measured (Figure 5).

(d) The time constant of the exponential decay curve fit to the maximal points during the muscular contraction period in the BFT (x^d): All maximal values between the first and last maximal values exceeding the MARS in a cycle were extracted as $\{x_m(t)\}$ and fit to the exponential decay curve $\hat{x}_m(t) = C\exp[-x^d t]$. On a semi-log graph, the time constant (x^d) was estimated using the mean least square method, which minimized the sum of the squared residuals;

$$L = \sum_t \{\log \hat{x}_m(t) - \log x_m(t)\}^2 \quad (2)$$

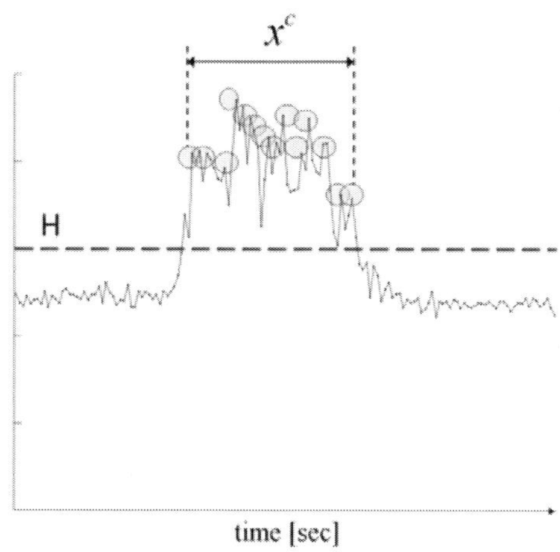

Figure 5. A series of maximal values of the ARS during the muscular contraction periods in the BFT that were extracted by our mathematical algorithm of the sensor output signal evaluation system.

In order to estimate the time constant (x^d), the following simultaneous equation should be solved.

$$\frac{\partial L}{\partial \log C} = 0, \frac{\partial L}{\partial x^d} = 0 \quad (3)$$

The numerical sequences of the 4 measurement parameters were determined at a repetition number of 6. The relationship between the age (z) of the subjects who had undergone sEMG and the value $x^i(z)$ (i = a,b,c,d) estimated in the 5th cycle was statistically examined to evaluate correlations between each measurement parameter and age (Appendix).

Practical Study of the SOSE System

The numerical sequences of each of the measurement parameters at a repetition number of 6 were obtained by sEMG performed during BFT. The relationship between the age (z) of the subjects who had undergone sEMG and the value $x^i(z)$ (i = a,b,c,d) was examined in 5th cycle. Figure 6 shows the $x^i(z)$ of all 50 subjects. The linear regression analysis using the least-square method, demonstrated that the coefficients by which age was multiplied were 0.061, -0.099, -0.004, and -0.010 for (a), (b), (c), and (d), respectively, and the parameters, except for (a), decreased with age. Since the linear regression coefficients varied with the measurement parameters, correlations between these parameters and age could not be judged using only the coefficients by which age (z) was multiplied. When using the t-test to evaluate the null hypothesis ($b\square = 0$) for the regression coefficient ($b\square$), the test values (A.3) were 1.105, 0.238, 1.621, and 3.245 for (a), (b), (c), and (d), respectively, and the only parameter exceeding $t_{48}(0.975)$ was the time constant of the exponential decay curve fit to the maximal points of the muscular contraction period in the BFT (x^d). We examined correlations between the parameters of the ARS and age. Regression equations (A.1) for each parameter (i = a,b,c,d) were determined, and the null hypothesis ($b\square = 0$) for the regression coefficient ($b\square$) was examined using the t-test. Since the test value (A.3) was larger than the two-sided 5% point, t_{48} (0.975), in the t distribution with a latitude of 48, the null hypothesis was rejected in the case of i = d. Therefore, the time constant of the exponential decay curve fit to the maximal points during the continuous muscular contraction period (x^d) is significantly dependant on age ($p<0.05$).

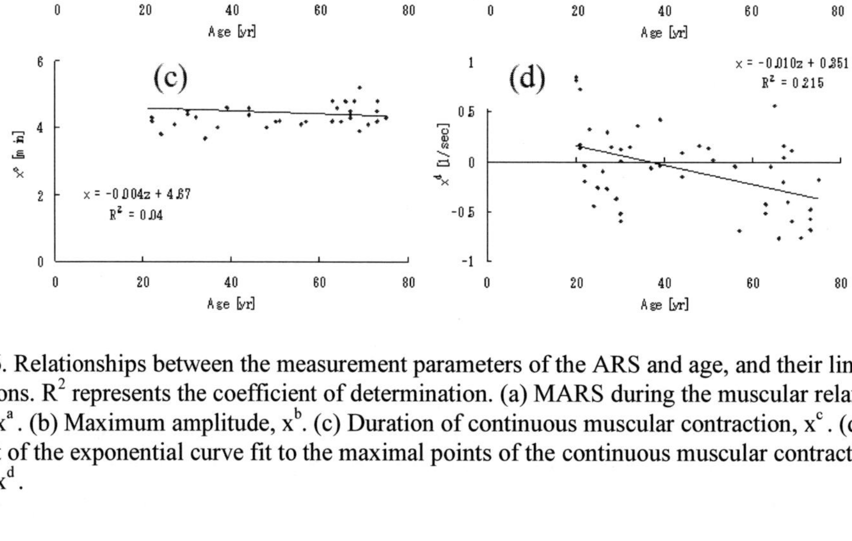

Figure 6. Relationships between the measurement parameters of the ARS and age, and their linear regressions. R^2 represents the coefficient of determination. (a) MARS during the muscular relaxation period, x^a. (b) Maximum amplitude, x^b. (c) Duration of continuous muscular contraction, x^c. (d) Time constant of the exponential curve fit to the maximal points of the continuous muscular contraction period, x^d.

Problem

The analysis of sEMG data is generally performed by the fast Fourier transformation (FFT), which is a linear analytical method. A Fourier series expansion of the function $f(t)$, showing target levels (instruction signals) for BFT, is possible, and the following expansion equation (Matsumoto and Miyahara, 1990) is useful for evaluating the differences between the ARS and the rectangular waves:

$$f(t) = 1 + \sum_{k=1}^{\infty} \frac{2}{k\pi} \{1 + (-1)^{k+1}\} \sin \frac{2\pi k}{T} t \tag{4}$$

Higher-order terms (high-frequency components) are included in this expansion equation, but the coefficients are small due to the presence of the order in the denominator. Accordingly, the high-frequency power was considered to be theoretically irrelevant for the evaluation shown in Eq. (4). Since muscular conditions always vary, signals should be regarded as non-steady (Beyer, 1987). Since a spectral estimation by the Fourier analysis is based on the assumption that the signals to be analyzed are steady and linear, this linear analysis of sEMG data is inappropriate.

In sEMG, a very large number of MU action potential waves are superimposed, and the activity states of whole muscles are observed by this method (Yoshida et al., 2004). Therefore, sEMG should be considered nonlinear, or more generally, sEMG shows a time series produced by stochastic processes. Recently, it has been recognized that sEMG data can be examined by nonlinear analytical methods, such as the recurrence plot and the Wayland algorithm (Yoshida et al., 2004; Takada et al, 2006c). However, the measurement parameters used in the present study, such as the time constant of the exponential decay curve fit to the maximal points of the continuous muscular contraction period (x^d), are used as a linear analytical method for sEMG. In the next section, we discuss the reason why we have succeeded in findings a linear index showing a correlation with age.

Solution & Recommendations

The complexity of the bio-signal or the degree of visible determinism generating those signals can be measured by our Double-Wayland algorithm (takada et al, 2006a), which is introduced in this section.

Double-Wayland Algorithm

The translation error is a statistical index that measures the smoothness of flow in an attractor generating a time series. In addition, randomness can be evaluated by the Double-Wayland algorithm by comparing the translation errors in the temporal differences of the time series (differenced time series) with the results of the Wayland algorithm in each embedding space (Wayland et al., 1993).

An attractor is reconstructed from a time series. The attractor is constructed by means of embedding the time series data proposed by Takens (1981) in the phase space. Embedding is a method that draws an orbit in phase space supposing a vector whose elements are the values for when the time elapses from t to Δt, 2Δt, …, (N-1) Δt as a point in N dimensional phase space (embedding space). N and Δt are referred to as the embedding dimension and the sampling time, respectively. The delay coordinates $\{\mathbf{x}(t)\}$ can reconstruct a continuous trajectory without crossing into an embedding space that has a high dimension. If we only resample the time series at every delay time τ when the auto-correlation coefficient $\rho(\tau)$ is regarded as zero, components of the delay coordinate

$$\mathbf{x} = (x(t) \quad x(t+\tau) \quad \cdots \quad x(t+(N-1)\tau))$$

cannot linearly correlate with each other. In this study, the auto-correlation function $\rho(t)$ was estimated from the time series data (Matsumoto et al., 2002) and regarded as zero when ρ(t) decreased below $1/e \cong 0.37$ for the first time ($t \geq 0$).

The Wayland algorithm assumes that the difference vectors $\mathbf{v}(t) = \mathbf{x}(t+\tau) - \mathbf{x}(t)$ in the embedding space characterize the nonlinear variations of the trajectories and estimate the translation error in an m-dimensional embedding space ($m = 1, 2, \ldots, 10$). Here, τ was estimated at 73-76 times the sampling time. A linear correlation between adjacent vectors $\mathbf{x}(t)$ and $\mathbf{x}(t+\tau)$ is eliminated by resampling the time series with respect to each embedding delay τ.

(i) A series of delay coordinate vectors $\{\mathbf{x}(t)\}$ is embedded in each space.
(ii) M onset periods t_0 are randomly selected.
(iii) The values of

$$E_{\text{trans}}(t_0) = \frac{1}{K+1}\sum_{i=0}^{K}\frac{\left|\mathbf{v}(t_i)-\overline{\mathbf{v}}\right|}{\left|\overline{\mathbf{v}}\right|} \tag{5}$$

are standardized by the average of the difference vectors at $K+1$ points $\{\mathbf{x}(t_i)\}_{i=0}^{K}$.

$$\overline{\mathbf{v}} = \frac{1}{K+1}\sum_{i=0}^{K}\mathbf{v}(t_i) \tag{6}$$

is obtained at every onset period, where the K points nearest to $\mathbf{x}(t_0)$ are selected as $\{\mathbf{x}(t_i)\}_{i=0}^{K}$.

(iv) The median of the M values of Eq. (5) is extracted.
(v) Q medians are obtained by repeating the above steps. The translation error E_{trans} is estimated by the expectation value of these Q medians.

The Double-Wayland algorithm includes the following additional steps.

(vi) Translation errors, E_{trans}', are derived from temporal differences in the time series data (differenced time series) $\{\mathbf{x}(t+\tau) - \mathbf{x}(t)\}$ by the Wayland algorithm outlined above.

(vii) If a differential equation system that included stochastic factors was the generator of the time series, the flow would not be smooth. In such a case, a significantly higher number of translation errors might be estimated in the last step than in step (v).

In this study, we set the conditions of the coefficients *M*, *K*, and *Q* to be 51, 3, and 10, respectively (Wayland et al., 1993).

If a time series is produced from a chaos process, the translation vectors point in almost the same direction unless the time implementation τ is too large, since deterministic aspects remain in time development. The minimum translation error would be estimated in such an embedding space that has no false intersection along the orbit and best reflects the degree of freedom. Hereby, the optimum embedding dimension to capture the chaos process can be obtained.

The differenced time series produced in the stochastic process often reconstitutes an indifferentiable orbit in embedding space. This indicates that the translation error estimated from the differenced time series exceeds the translation error estimated from the time series data. Accordingly, we weighed the translation error estimated from the time series data against the error estimated from the differenced time series in *m* dimensional phase space.

In general, the threshold of the translation error for classifying the time series data as deterministic or stochastic is 0.5, which is half of the translation error resulting from a random walk (Matsumoto et al., 2002). The abovementioned E_{trans} is compared with the translation error (E_{trans}') estimated from the sequences of the differenced time series.

Non-linear Analysis of the sEMG in the BFT

Using the Double-Wayland algorithm, translation errors were estimated from the sEMG measured during a continuous muscle contraction period and during BFT. We compared the translation errors, E_{trans} and E_{trans}', in each embedding space (Table 1). Intermittent muscle contractions during BFT resulted in fewer translation errors than estimated by the difference between the EMGs of the younger subjects. E_{trans}' would be less than E_{trans} if the degree of determinism involved in the generator was reduced. A rectangular wave as a teacher signal may reduce the nonlinearity involved in the generator of sEMG for young subjects. Moreover, we employed the surrogate data method to ascertain the cause of the correlation between age and a linear index for the ARS. According to the Fourier shuffle algorithm, 20 surrogate sequences were generated from each ARS during the 2 s continuous muscle contraction period and the 2 s of BFT. Using the Wayland algorithm, translation errors were estimated from the surrogate sequences. The embedding delay was estimated and is shown in Table 2. A significant difference was observed between the number of translation errors, E_{trans}', which were estimated from the ARS and the surrogate data during the continuous muscle contraction period ($p < 0.01$). E_{trans}' was did changed during the BFT (Table 3). These results demonstrate that could enhance the linearity in the generation of sEMG.

Table 1. Results of the calculations involved in sEMG using the Double-Wayland algorithm

(a)					
Embedding space	1	2	3	4	5
E_{trans}	1.05 ± 0.09	1.36 ± 0.08	1.39 ± 0.07	1.23 ± 0.08	1.17 ± 0.06
E_{trans}'	0.95 ±0.03	0.98 ± 0.05	1.03 ± 0.03	0.98 ± 0.03	0.97 ± 0.03
Embedding space	6	7	8	9	10
E_{trans}	1.19 ± 0.05	1.16 ± 0.09	1.14 ± 0.07	1.11 ± 0.05	0.99 ± 0.05
E_{trans}'	1.01 ± 0.04	1.06 ± 0.03	1.06 ± 0.03	1.08 ± 0.04	0.99 ± 0.03
(b)					
Embedding space	1	2	3	4	5
E_{trans}	0.90 ± 0.05	0.93 ± 0.04	0.92 ± 0.02	0.91 ± 0.02	0.98 ± 0.03
E_{trans}'	0.55 ± 0.04	0.49 ± 0.03	0.38 ± 0.01	0.38 ± 0.01	0.34 ± 0.01
Embedding space	6	7	8	9	10
E_{trans}	0.97 ± 0.03	0.98 ± 0.02	1.00 ± 0.02	1.04 ± 0.02	1.04 ± 0.01
E_{trans}'	0.34 ± 0.01	0.33 ± 0.00	0.33 ± 0.00	0.34 ± 0.00	0.35 ± 0.00

Table 2. Embedding delay used in Table 1

	Continuous muscle contraction period	BFT
ARS	0.16 ± 0.00 s	0.38 ± 0.00 s
Surrogate data of ARS	0.16 ± 0.01 s	0.17 ± 0.03 s

Table 3. Result of the surrogate data analysis

	Continuous muscle contraction period	BFT
ARS	0.87 ± 0.06 s	0.88 ± 0.09 s
Surrogate data of ARS	0.93 ± 0.07 s	0.94 ± 0.07 s

The decline in the number of translation errors, E_{trans}', was not always seen in the middle-aged and the elderly. Poor muscular control might enhance the instability of the temporal variations involved in the ARS, which should be maintained as a constant during a muscular contraction in BFT. The relationship between age and the value of translation errors, E_{trans}', will be investigated by our team in future.

Applicability

In recent times, there has been increasing focus on the rapid reduction of the muscles required for bending the hip joint during walking with age. Atrophy of the flexor muscles has been implicated in falling in the elderly. We examined the ARS of the femoral rectus muscles of the dominant leg during BFT. A reduction in muscular control could also be detected in sEMGs of the perineal muscles obtained during BFT using the time constant (Takada et al., 2006a). Moreover, statistical analysis indicated that it was necessary to include the time constant of the exponential decay curve fit to the maximal points during prolonged muscular contraction to evaluate changes with age using ARS during BFT for the flexor muscles around the hip joint (Takada et al., 2009) (Takada et al., 2010; Takada et al., in press).

The efficacy in the abovementioned linear index was evaluated using our non-linear analysis method (takada et al., 2006b) and has been previously described (Takada et al., 2011a). We also confirmed the stationary nature of ARS during the muscle contraction period.

We believe that the SOSE system can be applied to various fields in conjunction with other new technologies. For instance, we are now examining whether the 3D device for training ciliary muscles reduces visual fatigue or pseudomyopia. The BFT of the muscles of mastication and the soleus will also be evaluated using this device to prevent adiposis and economy class syndrome, respectively.

Ciliary Muscles

We are now examining whether the 3D device for training ciliary muscles, which control the lens' accommodation, reduces visual fatigue and pseudomyopia (Takada et al., 2011b). A new 3D movie technique produced by Olympus Visual Communications, Ltd. was incorporated in this device (Gaarder and Montgomery, 1981).

We assume that it is possible to improve an abnormal accommodative function of the lens by activating the muscles by alternately repeating negative and positive accommodation. By improving the abnormal accommodative function, we can improve or prevent these vision problems. We call this operation "accommodation training." In Japan, an apparatus was developed by Kobayashi (1994). The objective of this apparatus is to recover visual acuity. This apparatus works by using a Landolt ring drawn on a flat plate that moves back and forth over a distance of 2 m in order to encourage alternately repeating negative and positive accommodation in the observers. However, a large space was required to employ the accommodation training with the use of this apparatus. On the other hand, the Eyesight-Recovering Stereoscopic Movie System is commonly known as "Dr. Rex." In the Dr. Rex, an LCD displaying stereoscopic videos and the visual acuity recovery device equipped with liquid crystal shutter eyeglasses. Dr. Rex Eye Care Program contains some stereoscopic video contents that simulate near and distant visual conditions (Figure 7). Alternately displaying the videos on the LCD and device at appropriate intervals is expected to improve and prevent myopia, presbiopia, and visual fatigue. The abnormal contraction of ciliary muscles due to the performance of a near-visual task for several hours causes various vision problems such as asthenopia and visual loss. However, these problems can be resolved by activating the muscles by alternately repeating negative and positive accommodation. We have verified the effect of accommodation training that uses the strategy of presenting a stereoscopic movie to myopic youth and measuring the spherical diopter (SPH), visual acuity (far/near vision), and subjective index of asthenopia obtained using a visual analog scale (VAS) (Takada et al., 2011b). The results of subjective evaluations before (pre) and after (post) viewing the stereoscopic videos were compared using the Wilcoxon signed ranks test, where the significance level p was set to be 0.05.

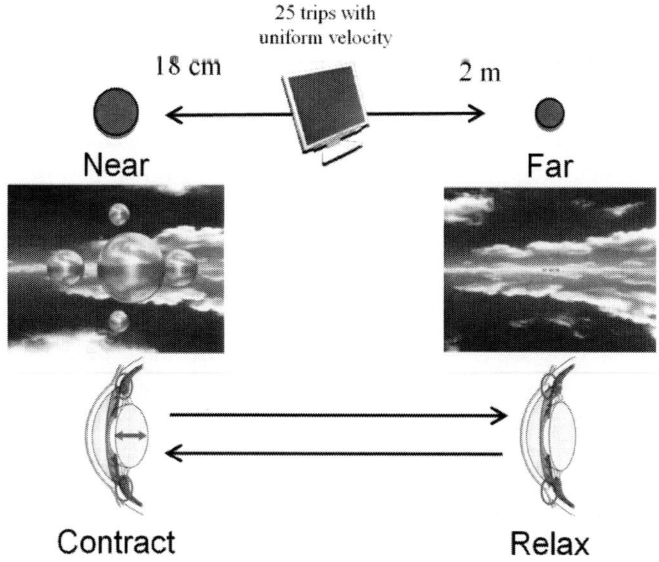

Figure 7. Schematic of the Dr. Rex Eye Care Program.

Soleus Muscles

The economy syndrome is also observed in refugees; hence, its evaluation is pertinent to relief efforts aimed at areas devastated by a massive earthquake. The muscle pump is considered a countermeasure and is expected to prevent bloodstream stagnation and the generation of atropic thrombosis. The bloodstream stagnation is also regarded as a problem in space deconditioning (Yamamoto et al., 2011). Using the SOSE system, we can both evaluate the preventive and remedial effects of BFT and increase its effectiveness.

Perineal Muscles

The number of elderly female patients who develop urinary incontinence (UI) is increasing yearly, which is caused by stress UI associated with dysfunction in the perineal muscles. Their quality of life is threatened by the disease. In the U.S.A., at least 13 million community-living adults and >50% of all residents in nursing facilities develop UI (Fantil et al., 1996).

The direct medical expenditures incurred for the care of these people is estimated to be >$15 billion annually, in addition to the $35.2 billion incurred annually for nursing home residents (Peek, 1995). There is a consensus that in most cases, behavioral treatment modalities including biofeedback should be used before invasive modalities such as surgery are employed.

Kegel (1948; 1951) was the first to use BFT for the treatment of UI, and it was observed that if the pelvic floor muscles are hypotonic, bladder suspension surgery is less effective for treating stress-related UI (Kegel, 1948; Kegel, 1951).

To improve the contractility of the pubococcygeus portion of the levator ani muscle, Kegel invented the pressure perineometer (Kegel, 1951).

Conclusion

Recently, there has been an increasing focus on the rapid reduction of the muscles that are required for bending the hip joint during walking with age. Atrophy of the flexor muscles has been implicated in falling in the elderly. In this study, we examined the ARS of the femoral rectus muscles during BFT of the dominant leg.

To this end, we developed parameters for the measurement of the shapes in the ARS, and evaluated the changes in these parameters as the muscles age.

A statistical analysis indicated that it was necessary to include the time constant of the exponential decay curve fit to the maximal points during prolonged muscular contraction to evaluate changes with age using the ARS during BFT. A reduction in the function of muscular control due to aging can be detected by performing sEMG during BFT using this time constant. Using our Double-Wayland algorithm, we have also confirmed the stationarity of the ARS during the muscle contraction period.

Acknowledgment

This work was supported in part by a ground-based study proposal for the fiscal year of 2005-2007 (17659189).

Appendix

The relationship between each of the above measurement parameters and age was examined. $x^i_j(z_j)$ of subject j ($j = 1,2,\cdots,50$) was plotted, and a linear regression analysis of these 50 points was performed by the least-square method (Matsumoto and Miyahara, 1990). The regression equation of each measurement parameter was determined.

$$x^i = \hat{a} + \hat{b} z \quad \text{(A.1)}$$

$$\text{s.t. } \hat{a} = \frac{1}{50}\left(\sum_{j=1}^{50} x^i_j - \hat{b}\sum_{j=1}^{50} z_j\right), \quad \text{(A.2.1)}$$

$$\hat{b} = \frac{1}{S_{zz}}\sum_{j=1}^{50} x^i_j\left(z_j - \frac{1}{50}\sum_{j=1}^{50} z_j\right). \ (i = \text{a, b, c, d}) \quad \text{(A.2.2)}$$

Here, S_{ZZ} denotes a variance of age. The dependence of each measurement parameter on age was statistically evaluated by a two-sided t-test with the null hypothesis that the regression coefficient $\hat{b} = 0$.

$$\left|\hat{b} - 0\right| \Big/ \sqrt{S_E / 48 S_{zz}} \quad \text{(A.3)}$$

If the above value is larger than $t_{48}(1-\alpha/2)$, the null hypothesis is rejected, and the measurement parameter is considered to be correlated with age (Shimizu and Takada, 2001). Here, S_E denotes the residual sum of squares by the least-square method, and $t_{48}(1-\alpha/2)$ represents the t distribution at a probability of $1-\alpha/2$ and a latitude of 48. In this study, since the significance level (α) was defined as 0.05, $t_{48}(1-\alpha/2)$ was approximately 2.010.

References

Aukee, P; Penttinen, J; Immonen, P; Airaksinen, O. Intravaginal surface EMG probe design test for urinary incontinence patients. *Acupunt. Electro-Ther. Res. Int. J.*, 2002 Vol.27, 37–44.

Basmajian, S. *An Anthology of Visual Poetry and Collage*, Toronto: Sober Minute Press; 1989.

Beyer, W.H. (eds.) *CRC Standard Mathematical Tables and Formulae.* 28th edition. Boca Raton, CRC Press; 1987.

De Luca, CJ. The Use of Surface Electromyography in Biomechanics. *Journal of Applied Biomechanics,* 1997 13, 135- 163.

Fantil, JA; Newman, DK; Colling, J. *Urinary incontinence in adults: Clinical Practice Guideline*, MI: University of Michigan Library, 1996.

Fisher, JP; Ogoh, S; Young, CN; Raven, PB; Fadel, PJ. Regulation of middle cerebral artery blood velocity during dynamic exercise in humans: influence of aging, *J Appl Phys*, 2008 vol. 105, 266–273.

Gaarder, KR; Montgomery, PS. *Clinical Biofeedback: A Procedural Manual for Behavioral Medicine*, London: Baltimore; 1981.

Gatchel, RJ; Price, KP. *Critical Applications of Biofeedback*, New York: Pergamon Press, 1979.

Jacobson, E. *Progressive Relaxation*, Chicago: University of Chicago Press; 1938.

Kegel, AH. Progressive resistance exercise in the functional restoration of the perineal muscles, Am J Obstet Gynecol, 1948 vol. 56, 238–248.

Kegel, AH. Physiologic therapy for urinary incontinence, *The Journal of the American Medical Association*, 1951 vol. 146, 915–917.

Kimura, J. *Electrodiagnosis in Diseases of Nerve and Muscles: Principles and Practice.* 2nd edition, Philadelphia: Oxford University Press, 1989, 209–304.

Kobayashi, S. Eye sight recovering apparatus. Japan Patent, 6-339501, 1994.

Kizuka, T; Masuda T; Kiryu T; Sadoyama T. *Practical Usage of Surface Electromyography.* Tokyo: Tokyo Denki University Press, 65–92, 2006.

Paulson, OB; Strandgaard, S; Edvinsson, L. Cerebral autoregulation, *Cerebrovasc Brain Metab Rev*, 1990 vol. 2, 161–192.

Matsumoto, H; Miyahara, Y. *Introduction to mathematical statistics*, Tokyo: Gakujutsu Tosho; 1999; 106-108.

Matsumoto, T; Tokunaga, R; Miyano, T; Tokuda, I. *Chaos and time series*, Tokyo: Baihukan; 2002; 49–64.

Peek, CJ. Title: A primer of biofeedback instrumentation. In: Schwartz, MS; Andrasik F, editors. *Title: Biofeedback*, New York: Guilford Press; 1995; 597–629.

Shimizu, Y; Takada, H. Verification of air temperature variation with form of potential, *Forma*, 2001 16(4), 339-356.

Shiozawa, T; Takada, H; Miyao, M. Sensor output signal evaluation system, Japan Patent, P2006-111387, 2006a.

Shiozawa, T; Takada, H; Miyao, M; Kawasaki, H. Propositions of evaluating indices of muscle performancs detected by using surface electromyography and evaluation of stability of the indices, *Proceedings of the 21th Symposium on Biological and Physiological Engineering 2006*, 2006b, 467-468.

Shiozawa, T; Takada, H; Miyao, M; Takada, M; Kawasaki, H; Watanabe, Y. Evaluation of muscle performances detected by using surface electromyography, *Japanese Journal of Ergonomics*, 2006c Vol.42, S440-S441.

Shiozawa, T; Takada, H; Miyao, M. Sensor output signal evaluation system, PCT Patent Publication No. WO, 2007/129452, 2007.

Takada, H; Watanabe, Y; Shiozawa, T; Takada, M; Gotoh, M; Miyao, M; Kawasaki, H. Quantitative evaluation of stability in surface electromyography for perineal muscle during biofeedback training, *Clin Neurophysiol*, 2006a vol.117, S280.

Takada, H; Morimoto, T; Tsunashima, H; Yamazaki, T; Hoshina, H; Miyao, M. Applications of double-wayland algorithm to detect anomalous signals. *Forma*, 2006b vol. 21, 159–167.

Takada, H; Shiozawa, T; Miyao, M; Nakayama, M; Kawasaki, H. Theoretical consideration to set the amplitude of teacher signal in the biofeedback training, *Proceedings of the 21th Symposium on Biological and Physiological Engineering 2006*, 2006c, 463-466.

Takada, H; Shiozawa, T; Takada, M; Iwase, S; Miyao, M. Evaluating indices of age-related muscle performance by using surface electromyography, *Proceedings of the 31st Annual International Conference of the IEEE Engineering in Medicine and Biology Society*, 2009, 6271–6275.

Takada, H; Shimozawa, T; Miyao, M; Matsuura, Y; Takada, M. Title: Consideration of indices to evaluate age-related muscle performance by using surface electromyography. In: Hamid, RA, editor. *Title: Advances in Computational Biology*, Boston: Springer; 2010; 585-591.

Takada, H; Matsuura, Y; Miyao, M; Shiozawa, T. Title: Nonlinear analysis of evaluation of age-related muscle performance using surface electromyography, In: Schwartz, M. Editor. *Title: EMG Methods for Evaluating Muscle and Nerve Function*, Rijeka(Croatia), InTech, 2011a, 91-106.

Takada, H; Matsuura, Y; Miyao, M. Title: Effectiveness of new technology to compose stereoscopic movies. In: Aamir, SM. Editor. *Title: Depth Map and 3D Imaging Applications: Algorithms and Technologies*. Hershey: IGI Global; 2011b.

Takada, H; Takada, M; Matsuura, Y; Miyao, M; Shiozawa, T. Study of surface electromyography and its indices to evaluate muscular control, *Forma*, in press.

Takens, F. Detecting strange attractors in turbulence, *Lecture Notes in Mathematics,* 1981 Vol.898, 366-381.

Tries, J; Eisman, E. Title: Urinary incontinence—evaluation and biofeedback treatment. In: Schwartz, MS, editor. *Title: Biofeedback a Practitionaer's Guide*. New York: Guilford Press; 1995; 597-629.

Wayland, R; Bromley, D; Pickett, D; Passamante, A. Recognizing determinism in a time series, *Physical Review Letters*, 1993 70(5), 580–582.

Yamamoto, T; Takada, H; Iwase, S; Sugenoya, J. Effects of graded load of artificial gravity on vestibulospinal and vestibule-ocular function, *Autonomic Nervous System*, 2011 Vol.47, 485–491.

Yoshida, H; Ujiie, H; Ishimura, K; Wada, M. The estimation of muscle fatigue using chaos analysis. *Journal of the Society of Biomechanisms,* 2004 vol. 28, 201–212.

In: Electromyography
Editor: Hiroki Takada

ISBN: 978-1- 62081-717-9

Chapter V

Surface Electromyographic Amplitude Normalization Methods: A Review

***Andreia S. P. Sousa*[1] *and João Manuel R. S. Tavares*[2]**

[1] Escola Superior de Tecnologia de Saúde do Porto, Área Científica de Fisioterapia,
Centro de Estudos de Movimento e Actividade Humana
Rua Valente Perfeito, 322, Vila Nova de Gaia, Portugal
Faculdade de Engenharia da Universidade do Porto
Rua Dr. Roberto Frias, s/n, Porto, Portugal
[2] Instituto de Engenharia
Mecânica e Gestão Industrial, Departamento de Engenharia Mecânica,
Faculdade de Engenharia, Universidade do Porto,
Rua Dr. Roberto Frias, s/n, Porto, Portugal

Abstract

The electromyogram is the summation of the motor unit action potentials occurring during contraction measured at a given electrode location. The voltage potential of the surface electromyographic signal detected by electrodes strongly depends on several factors, varying between individuals and also over time within an individual. Thus, the amplitude of the EMG signal itself is not useful in group comparisons, or to follow events over a long period of time. The fact that the recorded electromyographic amplitude is never absolute is mainly because impedance varies between the active muscle fibers and electrodes and its value is unknown. The EMG signal is highly variable and is dependent upon many factors. Thus, the amplitude of the temporally processed electromyography can only be used to assess short-term changes in the activity of a single muscle from the same individual when the electrode setup has not been altered. To allow comparison of activity between different muscles, across time, and between individuals, the EMG signal should be normalized, i.e. expressed in relation to a reference value obtained during standardized and reproducible conditions.

[1] E-mail: asp@estsp.ipp.pt.
[2] E-mail: tavares@fe.up.pt.

Notwithstanding the importance of electromyographic amplitude normalization, studies on functional activities, such as gait, do not seem to show a uniform methodology. Taking this into account, the main purpose of this chapter is to review and discuss different normalization procedures to relate the most appropriate method for specific situations, based on how the normalization method might influence data interpretation. In addition, this review supports the development of proper normalization procedures for biomechanical studies of functional activities like human gait.

Keywords: Biomechanics, electromyography, isometric actions, dynamic actions, isokinetic actions, human gait

Introduction

Electromyography (EMG) is unique in specifying muscle activation. Specifically, surface EMG is a convenient index of muscle excitation and allows a description of muscular patterns (Bouisset & Do, 2008). Analysis of amplitude modulation is usually performed with the signal envelope (rectification and low-pass filtering) or by estimation of the average rectified or root-mean-square value with a sliding window (Campanini, Merlo et al., 2007). However, absolute EMG amplitude values are not reliable, due to many factors which can influence them (Farina, Merletti et al., 2004). Variance of the estimate can be substantially reduced with special techniques, such as signal whitening and multichannel processing (Campanini, Merlo, et al., 2007). Nevertheless, the main limitation in the interpretation of EMG amplitude results not from processing algorithms but from the masking effects of unwanted factors.

The use of amplitude modulation for the assessment of relative muscle activation during movement relies on two main requirements: 1) EMG amplitude should be directly related to the level of excitation sent to the muscle from the spinal cord (Bonato, 2001), and 2) amplitude should not be influenced by factors other than the excitation level (Bonato, Roy et al., 2001). Both requirements are difficult to satisfy during dynamic contractions: Amplitude is not directly related to the excitation level because of amplitude cancellation (Farina, Merletti, et al., 2004). Moreover, the relation between amplitude and excitation level depends on the pattern of motor unit activation (Fuglevand, Winter et al., 1993), electrode location in relation to innervations zones and tendon regions, and crosstalk. In dynamic contractions, volume conductor properties (Mesin, Joubert et al., 2006) and the relative position of the electrodes with respect to muscle fibers may vary over time; therefore, amplitude may be additionally influenced by geometrical factors, in a subject- and muscle-specific way. Quantitative comparisons of patterns of EMG amplitude during movement across muscles or subjects should consequently require analysis of the possible confounding factors.

Importance of Normalization Procedures

The electromyogram is the summation of the motor unit action potentials occurring during the contraction measured at a given electrode location. This activity is often expressed in millivolts, but other units can be output by the acquisition device. EMG normalization is the process by which the electrical signal values of activity are expressed as a percentage of that muscle's activity during a calibrated test contraction (Lehman & McGill, 1999). Aiming to improve absolute EMG reliability and to provide an expression of relative muscle activation, the normalization of EMG data requires the use of a standardized and reliable reference value against which experimental data are measured (Burden, Trew et al., 2003).

The amplitude and frequency characteristics of the raw EMG acquired using surface electrodes has been shown to be sensitive to many intrinsic and extrinsic factors (DeLuca, 1997).

As such, the amplitude of the temporally processed EMG can only be used to assess short-term changes in the activity of a single muscle from the same individual when the electrode setup has not been altered (Mathiassen, 1997; Mathiassen, Winkel et al., 1995). To allow the comparison of activity between different muscles, across time, and between individuals, the EMG should be normalized (DeLuca, 1997; Knutson, Soderberg et al., 1994; Mathiassen, Winkel, et al., 1995; Mirka, 1991; Yang & Winter, 1984), i.e. expressed in relation to a reference value obtained during standardized and reproducible conditions (Mathiassen, Winkel, et al., 1995).

The fact that the acquired EMG amplitude is never absolute is mainly because the impedance varies between the active muscle fibers and electrodes and its value is unknown (Gerdle, Karlsson et al., 1999). The EMG is highly variable and is dependent upon electrode application and placement (Jensen, Vasseljen et al., 1993), perspiration and temperature (Winkel & Jørgensen, 1991), muscle fatigue (Hansson, Strömberg et al., 1992), contraction velocity and muscle length, cross talk from nearby muscles (McGill & Norman, 1986), activity in other synergists and antagonists (Mathiassen & Winkel, 1990), subcutaneous fat thickness, and slight variation in task execution (McGill, 1991), to name a few.

It would be impossible to control all these modulators of EMG amplitude in a clinical setting. Therefore, when comparing amplitude variables between measurements, normalization of some kind is required, i.e. the EMG signal is converted into a scale that is common to all measurement occurrences.

Normalization controls for the aforementioned variables and facilitates the comparison of EMG signals across muscles, between subjects, or between days for the same subject. By expressing the neural activity (EMG amplitude) as a percentage of the reference task, interpretation of the signal is moved into a framework of biological significance (Lehman & McGill, 1999).

Amplitude Normalization Methods

As already mentioned, because of the inherent variability of EMG signal, clinical interpretation of surface EMG requires the normalization of the EMG signal for physiological interpretation and for comparison between muscles and between subjects. Previous studies have used a number of different methods to produce reference EMG values for normalization purposes that can be repeated across participants and test days, including isometric, isokinetic and dynamic muscle actions (Burden, Trew, et al., 2003; Lehman & McGill, 1999; Yang & Winter, 1984), Figure 1.

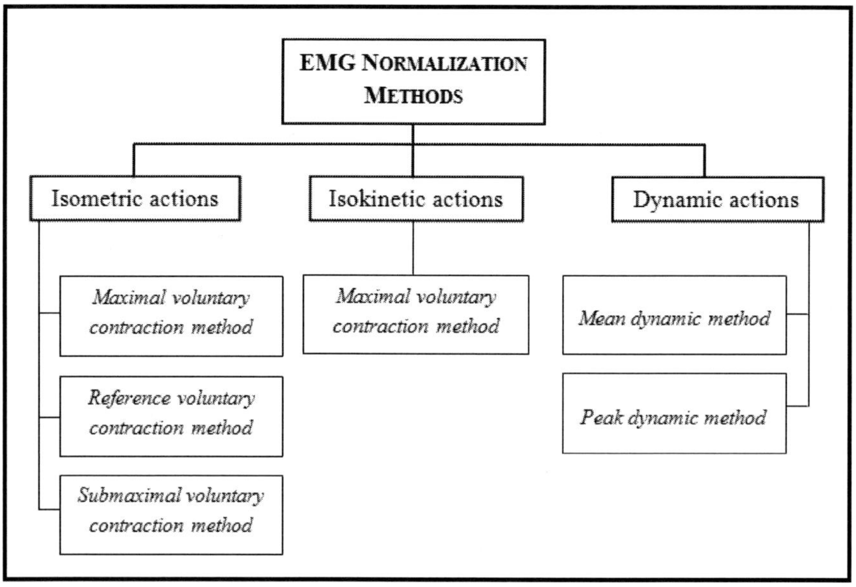

Figure 1. Usual electromyographic normalization methods.

A) Isometric Actions

Maximal and Submaximal Voluntary Contraction Methods

Typically, EMG is expressed as a percentage of the maximum neural drive acquired while a subject performs an isometric maximal voluntary contraction (MVC) of the desired muscle. This is perhaps the most powerful strategy for physiologic interpretation in healthy people. However, maximal effort contractions are not usually possible for older patients or for patients with symptoms. Also, acquiring maximal electrical activity is not always achieved during an effort involving maximal force generation (Lehman & McGill, 1999).

The use of MVC has several technical concerns, which have an impact on the validity and reliability of the normalization protocol, associated with isometric testing. These concerns include the inertial effects at the onset of the test, and the patient fatigue, posture and motivation. Furthermore, normalization is not a measure of muscular tension, but is a measure of muscular activation expressed as a percentage of activity relative to the subject's MVC (Soderberg, 1992). Therefore, the EMG from an isometric MVC may not represent the maximum activation capacity of the muscle either at lengths other than those at which the MVC was performed, or under non-isometric conditions, as was shown by (Mirka, 1991). Additionally, the other major limitation of using the EMG from an MVC as the denominator in the normalization equation concerns the poor reliability of EMG signal that has been reported from such contractions (Clarys, 2000; Perry, 1992; Yang & Winter, 1983).

In spite of the aforementioned limitations, maximal isometric muscle actions are the suggested method of normalizing by SENIAM and Kinesiology's guidelines and are the most widely employed normalization method (Burden, Trew, et al., 2003; DeLuca, 1997). Despite some studies demonstrating good EMG reliability between days (Hsu, Tang et al., 2002) and acceptable EMG reliability either between days or between weeks (Ball & Scurr, 2010), the majority of research has shown poor EMG reliability both within and between subjects and between sessions for isometric EMG levels of different muscles, particularly at maximal loads due to fatigue onset (Ball & Scurr, 2010; Bamman, Ingram et al., 1997; Heinonen, Sievänen et al., 1994; Yang & Winter, 1983), synergistic contribution and psychological factors (Enoka & Fuglevand, 1993; Miaki, Someya et al., 1999; Yang & Winter, 1983). Due to this instability of the EMG signal at near maximal levels, in (DeLuca, 1997) it is recommended that EMG amplitudes are normalized to force levels that are 80% of the maximum voluntary muscle action. Previous research has demonstrated that sub-maximal loads produced improved reliability between days compared to maximal loads for knee extensors and triceps (Rainoldi, Galardi et al., 1999; Yang & Winter, 1983). All the aforementioned methods provide an output that relates the task EMG to the EMG obtained during a particular standardized event and, as such, were termed as bioelectric normalizations in (Mathiassen, Winkel, et al., 1995). An alternative manner of normalization involves translating the EMG that forms the denominator of the equation in the isometric methods into a force or torque variable. Typically, the EMG is related to a maximal contraction, or a submaximal contraction at a known level of force. One purpose of such biomechanical normalization methods is to generate an estimate of the physical load on the muscle under investigation (Marras & Davis, 2001; Mathiassen, Winkel, et al., 1995).

Reference Voluntary Contraction Method

Controlled reference voluntary contractions (RVC) postures are interesting for clinical populations who are unable to attempt maximal efforts or who need an analogous controlled task for interpreting repeated tests. For example, standing upright holding 5 kg in the hands with the arms outstretched horizontally during each test session will produce a very similar low back moment day after day. Any change in un-normalized EMG amplitude could be due to any of the modulators and artifacts noted in the previous section. Any change in EMG amplitude (normalized to this RVC) indicates a true increase or decrease in the neural drive (Lehman & McGill, 1999).

B) Dynamic Muscle Actions

Peak Dynamic and Mean Dynamic Methods

Gait EMG signal was first normalized using a method that divided each point that constitutes the processed EMG by the peak value acquired from the same EMG. This method, subsequently referred to as the *peak dynamic method*, still appears to be popular among gait electromyographers (e.g. (Arendt-Nielsen, Graven-Nielsen et al., 1996; van Hedel, Tomatis et al., 2006)). In (Yang & Winter, 1984) a number of normalization methods are compared in an attempt to find the one which could provide a normal gait EMG template and, therefore, improve the use of electromyography as a diagnostic tool in gait analysis. Based on this rationale, the criterion for selecting the best method was the one that most reduced the inter-individual variability of the ensemble averaged EMG signal. The authors concluded that the *mean and peak dynamic methods* would help reduce the subject-specific and situation-specific conditions that may increase signal variance. They also pointed out that using these methods came at the expense of information inherent on the variance of the EMG signal. In (Ball & Scurr, 2010) it was found that squat jump and sprint provided reliable EMG amplitudes both between days and between weeks for all muscles of the triceps surae.

However, dynamic tasks such as reaction tests (Horstmann, Gollhofer et al., 1988), sub-maximal running, one-leg hopping, drop jumps (Gollhoferl, Horstmann et al., 1990) and walking (Kadaba, Ramakrishnan et al., 1989) have shown poor EMG reliability between testing sessions.

C) Isokinetic Actions

Electromyography amplitudes from an isokinetic muscle action have been proposed as an alternative to isometric muscle actions for EMG normalization to allow joint angle, torques and corresponding EMG amplitudes to be quantified (Kellis & Baltzopoulos, 1996; Mirka, 1991). Good EMG reliability has been shown between trials for isokinetic exercises for the knee extensors and flexors (Finucane, Rafeei et al., 1998; Larsson, 2003) and inappropriate reliability has been shown between isokinetic exercises for the triceps surae muscles (Ball & Scurr, 2010).

EMG Amplitude Normalization during Gait

Early investigations of dynamic tasks, including walking (Arsenault, Winter et al., 1986; Dubo, Peat et al., 1976), have used the EMG from an isometric MVC as the normalization reference value. However, it is generally recognized that the EMG from an isometric MVC is less reliable than the signal obtained from an isometric submaximal contraction (Yang & Winter, 1983), and that it might not represent the maximum activation capacity of the muscle (Enoka & Fuglevand, 1993). This has led to the evaluation and use of other reference values; in addition, some authors have expressed alternative aims for EMG normalization (Winter & Yack, 1987; Yang & Winter, 1983). As already mentioned, (Yang & Winter, 1984) compared four different normalization reference values to identify which one would result in the greatest reduction in inter-subject variability during walking. The use of either the mean or the peak linear envelope from the ensemble average of at least six strides reduced the inter-subject coefficient of variation in relation to the un-normalized data in all five lower limb muscles analyzed. In comparison, the inter-subject coefficient of variation was generally increased by using either 50% of the isometric MVC or the mean EMG per unit of isometric moment as the reference values. A reduced inter-subject coefficient of variation was also demonstrated for the biceps brachii during isotonic elbow flexions and extensions (Allison, Marshall et al., 1993) and for the gastrocnemius during a balancing task (Knutson, Soderberg, et al., 1994) by using the peak or mean ensemble value in comparison to the EMG from an isometric submaximal contraction (Allison, Marshall, et al., 1993) or MVC (Allison, Marshall, et al., 1993; Knutson, Soderberg, et al., 1994). Although the peak and mean ensemble methods are the only feasible ways of normalizing EMG signal from patients with neurologic disorders (Yang & Winter, 1984), such methods tend to produce a normal EMG template for a particular task and, therefore, may remove the true biological variation within a group (Allison, Marshall, et al., 1993; Knutson, Soderberg, et al., 1994). While the isometric MVC method is the only one that aims to reveal the percentage of the maximum activation capacity of the muscle required to perform a specific task (Yang & Winter, 1984), generally, the other methods mentioned above lead to changes in the un-normalized data as a consequence of variations in load and velocity of movement (Allison, Marshall, et al., 1993). In (Knutson, Soderberg, et al., 1994) the EMG activity of the gastrocnemius muscle was evaluated during gait using the MVC, mean dynamic method and peak dynamic method normalization in anterior cruciate ligament injured subjects. Data were compared statistically for the inter-class coefficient of variance (CV), variance ratio (VR) and intra-class coefficient of variance (ICC), being concluded that normalizing to MVC provided the most reproducible results based on the VR and ICC. However, this work did not identify how the normalization method might influence data interpretation and the justification for using the MVC method seems contradictory to that of (Yang & Winter, 1984) for rectus femoris, vastus lateralis, biceps femoris, tibialis anterior, and soleus muscles.

A) Mean Dynamic Method of Normalization of the EMG Signal during a Full Gait Cycle

The mean dynamic method represents an average of both quiet and active periods during the gait cycle. Therefore, it may be more susceptible to systems with a low signal noise ratio, or it may represent baseline noise in movements that cause very phasic activation. This method, depicted in Figure 2, is more conservative as the overall variability in the signal may be reduced at the expense of true changes in activation level (Benoit, Lamontagne et al., 2003).

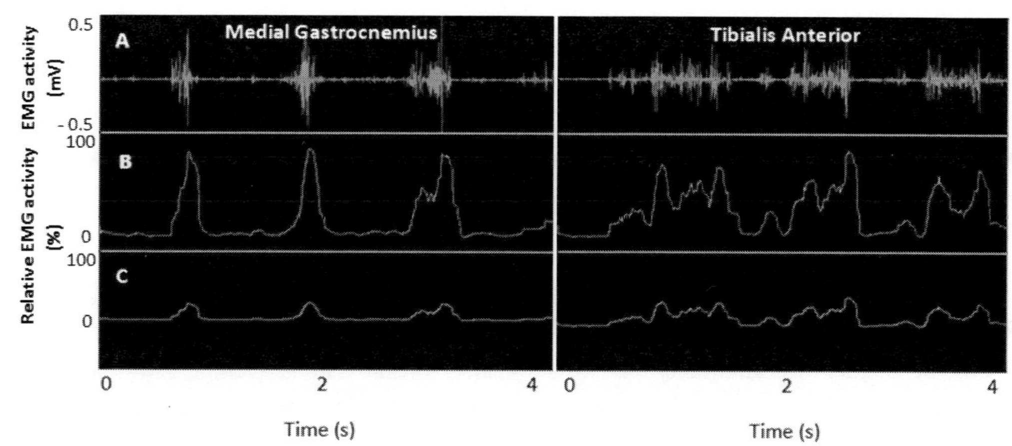

Figure 2. Raw EMG signal of medial gastrocnemius and tibialis anterior muscles obtained during gait at self-selected speed (A). The raw EMG signal was filtered and processed according to the root mean square (RMS) procedure and then normalized according to *mean dynamic* (B) and *peak dynamic* (C) methods.

B) Peak Dynamic Method of Normalization of the EMG Signal During a Full Gait Cycle

When representing the percentage of the peak dynamic method of EMG signal during repeated gait cycles (Figure 2), the procedure indicates the periods during the gait cycle at which the muscle is most active. However, it does not indicate the muscle's ability to activate. Therefore, the amount of activation cannot be related to any physiological measure and the patients' inability to contract the muscle due to pain inhibition, and altered neuromuscular performance, may not be observed (Benoit, Lamontagne, et al., 2003).

C) Isometric Maximal Voluntary Contraction Method

Evidence suggests that the isometric maximal voluntary contraction (MVC) method best represents isotonic contractions at various speeds (Burden & Bartlett, 1999) and, with modeling, can estimate muscle forces during gait. However, adding to the disadvantages already mentioned, normalizing to isometric contraction does not represent dynamic contraction. The advantage of this technique is that normalization is based on the patients' ability to contract the muscle. Yet, this ability to perform a MVC is greatly affected by pain, and when the pain is inhibited with local analgesia postoperatively, there is an increase in the patients' ability to contract voluntarily the quadriceps to a maximal level (Arvidsson, Eriksson et al., 1986). The influence of pain-induced muscle inhibition would probably only affect the data when normalized to the MVC method. On the other hand, if the subject was unable to contract the muscle maximally during the MVC protocol, the relative amount of activation required during a cyclical movement such as gait might be represented by a change in the amount of activation recorded, and not merely by changes in temporal parameters. Although additional methods exist, such as using interpolated-twitch techniques (Rudolph, Axe et al., 2001) and using torque measurements to model the force output of the various muscle groups, these may not provide useful clinical information for rehabilitation purposes.

All normalization methods exposed present advantages and limitations, Table 1. Normalization by the isometric of MVC is unreliable (DeLuca, 1997) since muscle contraction during gait is mostly isotonic (Winter & Scott, 1991). The isokinetic MVC method has been used as a method to simulate with a higher degree of comparability to muscle contractions during gait. However, when compared to the isometric MVC method, it did not always produce satisfactory results, especially if one considers that it is better to have lower CV and lower VR, which represents the intra- and inter-individual variability of the EMG profile (Burden, Trew, et al., 2003).

Another object of normalizing the EMG signal is to establish an average EMG profile to be a reliable template. Therefore, the peak dynamic method and the mean dynamic method have also been used (Winter and Yack, 1987; Yang and Winter, 1984), in addition to the two normalization methods referred above. Additionally, it has been reported that profiles obtained with these methods are close to one another, and that the mean method produces better results with respect to reliability, as already mentioned. However, it has also been noted that normalization by using the peak and mean methods, which do not use reference values obtained from reference exercises, intentionally removes the true biological variation within a normal group (Allison, Marshall, et al., 1993; Knutson, Soderberg, et al., 1994).

In (Nishijima, Kato et al., 2010), a different normalization method based on exercises under submaximal load (segment weight dynamic movement) is proposed. According to these authors, this method is as applicable as the isometric MVC method as a normalization method for establishing a gait EMG profile template.

Moreover, for all of the eight muscles studied, the gait EMG peak amplitudes were lower than those obtained from the reference exercises of the segment weight dynamic movement method. Therefore, at least in terms of muscular activity level, being able to carry out the reference exercises may serve as a criterion of a person having a sufficient muscular activity level required for walking.

In Figure 3, the results of different EMG amplitude normalization methods are presented for rectus femoris (RF) activity during terminal stance of gait at self-selected speed. To access the EMG activity during isometric and isokinetic MVC the subject was positioned in closed kinetic chain on a quadriceps chair, under the following criteria: (i) hip and knee at 90° flexion; (ii) stabilization of the torso, the pelvis, right below the anterior superior iliac spine, and thighs; (iii) resistance applied 3 cm above the malleoli; (iv) arms crossed over the chest. Isometric MVC of RF muscle was performed by reaching maximal force as rapidly as possible and maintaining it for 3 seconds.

Submaximal MVC was performed with 40% of isometric MVC and maintained for 3 seconds. Isokinetic MVC of the knee extensors was performed concentrically at 0.52 rad·s^{-1} interval up to 6.28 rad·s^{-1} between 90° and 0° of knee flexion. Reference contraction was obtained by asking the subject to hold a standardized load (3 kg). RF EMG activity during gait propulsion was expressed as a percentage of the peak RMS EMG from the isometric and isokinetic MVC, submaximal MVC and reference contraction.

Dynamic repetitive movement exercises under the load of the segment weight (segment weight dynamic movement exercise (SWDM)) of the quadriceps femoris was performed with the subject seated with legs dangling and performed knee extension from lower-limb-dangling position to knee-extended position. Each SWDM exercise was repeated 15 times at 30 rep/min using a metronome.

For each SWDM exercise, the peak amplitude during concentric contraction was measured in 12 trials, excluding the first 3 trials (where frequent EMG pattern variations were observed, probably due to the instability during initial periods of repetitive exercises), and the average value of 10 (excluding the highest and lowest values) was used as the 100% SWDM value. For mean dynamic method (MDM) and peak dynamic method (PDM), the RMS of EMG activity of propulsion was expressed as a percentage of the mean and the peak RMS of EMG activity of the intra-individual ensemble average,

$$X_{norm} = \frac{X - X_b}{X_{mean} - X_b} \tag{1}$$

and

$$X_{norm} = \frac{X - X_b}{X_{peak} - X_b}, \tag{2}$$

respectively, where X is the current value of the considered variable, X_{norm} is its normalized value, X_b is the baseline activity of RF muscle, X_{mean} and X_{peak} are the mean and maximum value observed along gait cycle.

As previously stated, the used normalization methods yield an output that is simply the ratio of the task EMG to the EMG used as the denominator in the normalization equation. As such, depending on the nature of the denominator, outputs from different normalization methods can differ in magnitude and pattern.

As depicted in Figure 3, different EMG normalization procedures lead to significant differences on the relative EMG amplitude developed during the activity assessed. Analyzing the normalized values of RF during propulsion it can be noted that this activity is extremely low when compared to the one obtained in maximal and submaximal contractions. However, this kind of normalization has a biological meaning since the values obtained during the activity are a percentage of the values obtained during maximal and submaximal contractions. The results show a higher magnitude of output from the MDM and PDM, which occurs as a result of using a smaller denominator in the normalization equation. Differences between these two methods are comprehensible taking into account the denominator values. Comparing MDM and PDM and the maximal and submaximal contraction methods, the first are more difficult to interpret as they are a percentage of the values obtained during the task. The RVC and SWDM normalization methods lead to relative values that are between the values obtained in the other methods and have more biological meaning than MDM and PDM.

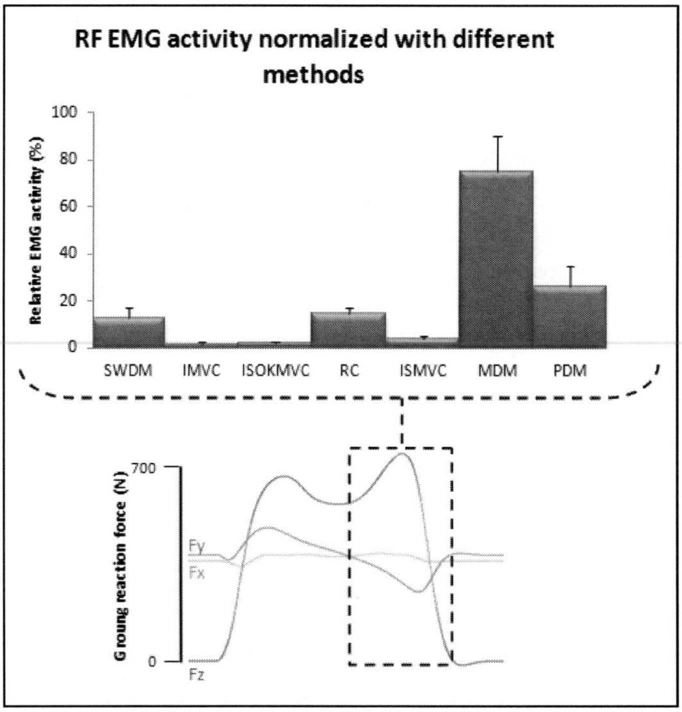

Figure 3. Relative EMG activity of RF obtained during terminal stance of gait at self-selected speed. Terminal stance was determinate throught ground reaction force trace in anteroposterior (Fy), mediolateral (Fx) and vertical (Fz) directions. Different normalization methods were used: segment weight dynamic movement (SWDM), isometric MVC (IMVC), isokinetic MVC (ISOKMVC), reference contraction (RC), isometric submaximal voluntary contraction (ISMVC), mean dynamic method (MDM) and peak dynamic method (PDM).

Effect of Normalization Method on Inter-Subject Variability of the EMG Signal

The use of normalization methods similar to the mean dynamic and peak dynamic methods has successfully reduced the inter-subject variability (Burden, Trew, et al., 2003; Winter & Yack, 1987; Yang & Winter, 1984).

In addition, there is strong evidence that using the dynamic mean normalization reduces the inter-subject variability in relation to other normalization methods (Allison, Marshall, et al., 1993; Burden & Bartlett, 1999; Burden, Trew, et al., 2003; Knutson, Soderberg, et al., 1994; Yang & Winter, 1984) and the un-normalized EMG (Allison, Marshall, et al., 1993; Burden & Bartlett, 1999; Yang & Winter, 1984).

Thus, if researchers or clinicians wish to retain the homogeneity of task-specific EMG signal for a group of individuals, they should avoid use of the peak dynamic method and, in particular, the mean dynamic normalization methods, as suggested elsewhere (Allison, Marshall, et al., 1993; Knutson, Soderberg, et al., 1994).

According to (Burden, Trew, et al., 2003), normalization by mean dynamic method resulted in slightly more homogeneous pattern of gait EMG signal than the peak dynamic method.

As to isokinetic maximal voluntary method, it should not be used in preference to the other methods, as is less reliable than un-normalized EMG signal or those normalized by the mean dynamic, peak dynamic or isometric maximal voluntary contraction methods (Burden, Trew, et al., 2003).

Ability of Normalization Method to Detect Changes in External Force

According to (Allison, Marshall, et al., 1993; Burden & Bartlett, 1999; Burden, Trew, et al., 2003), the isometric and isokinetic MVC methods reflect the increase in EMG that occurs in response to increments in external force.

Unlike the MVC methods, the dynamic mean and dynamic peak normalization methods are not designed to provide the percentage of the maximal activation capacity of the muscle required to perform the isotonic contractions.

Hence, it is unsurprising that the output of the mean dynamic normalization, and in particular the mean dynamic normalization methods, were unable to reflect the increase in EMG that occurred in response to the increase in force (Burden & Bartlett, 1999).

This disagrees with the findings of (Allison, Marshall, et al., 1993) stating that normalization methods using either the mean or the peak EMG from the ensemble average were able to distinguish between load and no-load conditions for the same muscle.

Table 1. Advantages, disadvantages/limitations and interpretation of normalization methods

Normalization method		Advantages	Disadvantages/Limitations	Data interpretation
Isometric method	*MVC method*	Perhaps the most powerful strategy for physiologic interpretation in healthy people.	Poor reliability. Is affected by inertial effects at the onset of the test, patient fatigue, patient posture, synergistic contribution, patient motivation, pain, neuro-muscle-skeletal dysfunctions and neurologic conditions. May not represent the maximum activation capacity in other lengths or under non-isometric conditions.	Represents the percentage of the maximum neural drive acquired while a subject performs an isometric MVC of the desired muscle. Any change in EMG amplitude indicates a true increase or decrease in the neural drive.
	Submaximal voluntary method	Resolves the instability of the EMG signal at near maximal levels.	Inter-subject coefficient of variation generally increases by using either 50% of the isometric MVC. Values can be lower than the obtained during the activity. Is affected by inertial effects at the onset of the test, patient fatigue, patient posture, synergistic contribution, patient motivation, pain, neuro-muscle-skeletal dysfunctions and neurologic conditions. Does not represent a dynamic contraction.	Percentage of the maximum neural drive acquired while a subject performs an isometric submaximal voluntary contraction of the desired muscle. Any change in EMG amplitude indicates a true increase or decrease in the neural drive.
	RVC method	Helpful for clinical populations who are unable to attempt maximal efforts or who need a similar controlled task for interpreting repeated tests.	Is affected by inertial effects at the onset of the test, patient fatigue, patient posture, synergistic contribution, pain, neuro-muscle-skeletal dysfunctions and neurologic conditions. Does not represent dynamic contraction.	Any change in normalized EMG amplitude indicates a true increase or decrease in the neural drive.

Normalization method		Advantages	Disadvantages/Limitations	Data interpretation
Isokinetic actions	*Isokinetic MVC method*	Has been used as a method to simulate with a higher degree of comparability muscle contractions obtained in dynamic activities.	Is less reliable than the other normalization methods.	Represents the percentage of the maximum neural drive acquired while a subject performs an isokinetic MVC of the desired muscle. Any change in EMG amplitude indicates a true increase or decrease in the neural drive.
Dynamic muscle actions	*Mean dynamic method*	Reduces the inter-subject variability in relation to other normalization methods. Helpful for clinical populations that are unable to attempt maximal efforts.	Tends to produce a normal EMG template for a particular task and, therefore, may remove the true biological variation within a group. It may be more susceptible to systems with a low signal to noise ratio or represent baseline noise in movements that cause very phasic activation. It does not give an indication of what this activity level means with respect to the muscle's ability to activate.	Represents a percentage of the average of both quiet and active periods during the activity.
	Peak dynamic method	Reduces the inter-subject variability in relation to other normalization methods. Helpful for clinical populations that are unable to attempt maximal efforts.	Tends to produce a normal EMG template for a particular task and, therefore, may remove the true biological variation within a group. It does not give an indication of what this activity level means with respect to the muscle's ability to activate.	Indicates at what periods during the activity the muscle is most active.

Conclusion

Different electromyography amplitude normalization methods have been described. We reviewed several studies that focus on comparing the different methods. Isometric and dynamic methods seem to be the most recommended. However, both present advantages and limitations, being important to understand clearly the purpose of the electromyographic study and the implications of the method adopted on the interpretation of the results attained. Table 1 summarizes the main topics discussed in this chapter concerning EMG signal normalization procedures and interpretation.

Acknowledgments

The first author would like to thank the PhD grant and the support and contribution from Instituto Politécnico do Porto (IPP) and Escola Superior de Tecnologia da Saúde (ESTSP), in Portugal.

References

Allison G. T., Marshall R. N. & Singer K. P. (1993). EMG signal amplitude normalization technique in stretch-shortening cycle movements. *Journal of Electromyography and Kinesiology*, 3 4, 236-244.

Arendt-Nielsen L., Graven-Nielsen T., Svarrer H. & Svensson P. (1996). The influence of low back pain on muscle activity and coordination during gait: a clinical and experimental study. *Pain*, 64 2, 231-240.

Arsenault A., Winter D. & Marteniuk R. (1986). Is there a 'normal' profile of EMG activity in gait? *Medical and Biological Engineering and Computing*, 24, 337-343.

Arvidsson I., Eriksson E., Knutsson E. & Arner S. (1986). Reduction of pain inhibition on voluntary muscle activation by epidural analgesia. *Orthopedics*, 9, 1415-1419.

Ball N. & Scurr J. (2010). An assessment of the reliability and standardisation of tests used to elicit reference muscular actions for electromyographical normalisation. *Journal of Electromyography and Kinesiology*, 20 1, 81-88.

Bamman M. M., Ingram S. G., Caruso J. F. & Greenisen M. C. (1997). Evaluation of Surface Electromyography During Maximal Voluntary Contraction. *The Journal of Strength & Conditioning Research*, 11 2, 68-72.

Benoit D. L., Lamontagne M., Cerulli G. & Liti A. (2003). The clinical significance of electromyography normalisation techniques in subjects with anterior cruciate ligament injury during treadmill walking. *Gait & Posture*, 18 2, 56-63.

Bonato P. (2001). Recent advancements in the analysis of dynamic EMG data. *IEEE Engineering In Medicine And Biology Magazine: The Quarterly Magazine Of The Engineering In Medicine & Biology Society*, 20 6, 29.

Bonato P., Roy S. H., Knaflitz M. & de Luca C. J. (2001). Time-frequency parameters of the surface myoelectric signal for assessing muscle fatigue during cyclic dynamic contractions. *IEEE Transactions on Biomedical Engineering*, 48 7, 745-753.

Bouisset S. & Do M. C. (2008). Posture, dynamic stability, and voluntary movement. *Neurophysiologie Clinique/Clinical Neurophysiology*, 38 6, 345-362.

Burden A. & Bartlett R. (1999). Normalisation of EMG amplitude: an evaluation and comparison of old and new methods. *Medical Engineering & Physics*, 21 4, 247-257.

Burden A. M., Trew M. & Baltzopoulos V. (2003). Normalisation of gait EMGs: a re-examination. *Journal of Electromyography and Kinesiology*, 13 6, 519-532.

Campanini I., Merlo A., Degola P., Merletti R., Vezzosi G. & Farina D. (2007). Effect of electrode location on EMG signal envelope in leg muscles during gait. *Journal of Electromyography and Kinesiology*, 17 4, 515-526.

Clarys J. P. (2000). Electromyography in sports and occupational settings: an update of its limits and possibilities. *Ergonomics*, 43 10, 1750 - 1762.

DeLuca C. (1997). The Use of Surface Electromiography in Biomechanics. *Journal of Applied Biomechanics*, 13 2, 135-163.

Dubo H., Peat M., Winter D., Quanbury A., Hobson D., Steinke T., et al. (1976). Electromyographic temporal analysis of normal gait: normal human locomotion. *Archives of Physical Therapy Medicine and Rehabilitation*, 57, 415-420.

Enoka R. & Fuglevand A. (1993). Neuromuscular basis of the maximum voluntary force capacity of muscle. In M. Grabiner (Ed.), *Current issues in biomechanics* (pp. 215-235). Champaign: Human Kinetics.

Farina D., Merletti R. & Enoka R. (2004). The extraction of neural stategies from surface EMG. *Journal of Applied Physiology*, 96, 1486-1495.

Finucane S. D. G., Rafeei T., Kues J., Lamb R. L. & Mayhew T. P. (1998). Reproducibility of electromyographic recordings of submaximal concentric and eccentric muscle contractions in humans. *Electroencephalography and Clinical Neurophysiology/ Electromyography and Motor Control*, 109 4, 290-296.

Fuglevand A. J., Winter D. A. & Patla A. E. (1993). Models of recruitment and rate coding organization in motor-unit pools. *Journal of Neurophysiology*, 70 6, 2470-2488.

Gerdle B., Karlsson S., Day S. & Djupsjobacka M. (1999). *Acquisition, processing and analysis of the surface electromyogram: Modern techniques in neuroscience*. Berlin: Springer.

Gollhoferl A., Horstmann G., Schmidtbleicher D. & Schönthall D. (1990). Reproducibility of electromyographic patterns in stretch-shortening type contractions. *European Journal of Applied Physiology and Occupational Physiology*, 60 1, 7-14.

Hansson G.-Å., Strömberg U., Larsson B., Ohlsson K., Balogh I. & Moritz U. (1992). Electromyographic fatigue in neck/shoulder muscles and endurance in women with repetitive work. *Ergonomics*, 35 11, 1341 - 1352.

Heinonen A., Sievänen H., Viitasalo J., Pasanen M., Oja P. & Vuori I. (1994). Reproducibility of computer measurement of maximal isometric strength and electromyography in sedentary middle-aged women. *European Journal of Applied Physiology and Occupational Physiology*, 68 4, 310-314.

Horstmann G. A., Gollhofer A. & Dietz V. (1988). Reproducibility and adaptation of the EMG responses of the lower leg following perturbations of upright stance. *Electroencephalography and Clinical Neurophysiology*, 70 5, 447-452.

Hsu A.-L., Tang P.-F. & Jan M.-H. (2002). Test-retest reliability of isokinetic muscle strength of the lower extremities in patients with stroke. *Archives of Physical Medicine and Rehabilitation*, 83 8, 1130-1137.

Jensen C., Vasseljen O. & Westgaard R. (1993). The influence of electrode position on bipolar surface electromyogram recordings of the upper trapezius muscle. *European Journal of Applied Physiology and Occupational Physiology*, 67 3, 266-273.

Kadaba M. P., Ramakrishnan H. K., Wootten M. E., Gainey J., Gorton G. & Cochran G. V. B. (1989). Repeatability of kinematic, kinetic, and electromyographic data in normal adult gait. *Journal of Orthopaedic Research*, 7 6, 849-860.

Kellis E. & Baltzopoulos V. (1996). The effects of normalization method on antagonistic activity patterns during eccentric and concentric isokinetic knee extension and flexion. *Journal of Electromyography and Kinesiology*, 6 4, 235-245.

Knutson L. M., Soderberg G. L., Ballantyne B. T. & Clarke W. R. (1994). A study of various normalization procedures for within day electromyographic data. *Journal of Electromyography and Kinesiology*, 4 1, 47-59.

Larsson B. K., S; Erikson, M; Glerdle, B; (2003). Test-retest reliability of EMG and peak torque during repetitive maximum concentric knee extensions. *Journal of Electromiography and Kinesiology*, 13 3, 281-287.

Lehman G. & McGill S. (1999). The Importance of Normalization in the Interpretation of Surface Electromyography:A Proof of Principle. *Journal of Manipulative and Physiological Therapeutics*, 22 7, 369-370.

Marras W. S. & Davis K. G. (2001). A non-MVC EMG normalization technique for the trunk musculature: Part 1. Method development. *Journal of Electromyography and Kinesiology*, 11 1, 1-9.

Mathiassen S. & Winkel J. (1990). Electromyographic activity in the shoulder-neck region according to arm position and glenohumeral torque. *European Journal of Applied Physiology and Occupational Physiology*, 61 5, 370-379.

Mathiassen S. E. (1997). *A checklist for normalisation of surface EMG amplitude.* Paper presented at the Proceedings of the Second General SENIAM Workshop Chapter 2, Stockholm, Sweden.

Mathiassen S. E., Winkel J. & Hägg G. M. (1995). Normalization of surface EMG amplitude from the upper trapezius muscle in ergonomic studies -- A review. *Journal of Electromyography and Kinesiology*, 5 4, 197-226.

McGill S. & Norman R. (1986). Partitioning of the L4/L5 dynamic moment into disc, ligamentous, and muscular components during lifting. *Spine*, 11, 666-678.

McGill S. M. (1991). Electromyographic activity of the abdominal and low back musculature during the generation of isometric and dynamic axial trunk torque: Implications for lumbar mechanics. *Journal of Orthopaedic Research*, 9 1, 91-103.

Mesin L., Joubert M., Hanekom T., Merletti R. & Farina D. (2006). A finite element model for describing the effect of muscle shortening on surface EMG. *IEEE Transactions on Biomedical Engineering*, 53, 593-600.

Miaki H., Someya F. & Tachino K. (1999). A comparison of electrical activity in the triceps surae at maximum isometric contraction with the knee and ankle at various angles. *European Journal of Applied Physiology and Occupational Physiology*, 80 3, 185-191.

Mirka G. A. (1991). The quantification of EMG normalization error. *Ergonomics*, 34 3, 343 - 352.

Nishijima Y., Kato T., Yoshizawa M., Miyashita M. & Iida H. (2010). Application of the segment weight dynamic movement method to the normalization of gait EMG amplitude. *Journal of Electromyography and Kinesiology*, 20 3, 550-557.

Perry J. (1992). *Gait Analysis: Normal and Pathological Gait.* Thorofare, NJ: Slack Incorporated.

Rainoldi A., Galardi G., Maderna L., Comi G., Lo Conte L. & Merletti R. (1999). Repeatability of surface EMG variables during voluntary isometric contractions of the biceps brachii muscle. *Journal of Electromyography and Kinesiology*, 9 2, 105-119.

Rudolph K. S., Axe M. J., Buchanan T. S., Scholz J. P. & Snyder-Mackler L. (2001). Dynamic stability in the anterior cruciate ligament deficient knee. *Knee Surgery, Sports Traumatology, Arthroscopy*, 9 2, 62-71.

Soderberg G. (1992). *Selected Topics in Surface Electromiography for Use in the Occupational Setting: Expert Perspectives.* Atlanta, GA: DHHS (NIOSH) Publication.

van Hedel H., Tomatis L. & Muller R. (2006). Modulation of leg muscle activity and gait kinematics by walking speed and bodyweight unloading. *Gait Posture*, 24, 35-45.

Winkel J. & Jørgensen K. (1991). Significance of skin temperature changes in surface electromyography. *European Journal of Applied Physiology and Occupational Physiology*, 63 5, 345-348.

Winter A. & Yack H. (1987). EMG profiles during normal walking: stride-to-stride and inter-subject variability. *Electromyography and Clinical Neurophysiology*, 67, 402-411.

Winter D. & Scott S. (1991). Technique for Interpretation of Electromyography for Concentric and Eccentric Contractions in Gait. *Journal of Electromyography and Kinesiology*, 1 4, 263-269.

Yang J. & Winter D. (1983). Electromyography reliability in maximal and submaximal isometric contractions. *Archives of Physical Medicine and Rehabilitation*, 64, 417-420.

Yang J. & Winter D. (1984). Electromyographic amplitude normalization methods: Improving their sensitivity as diagnostic tools in gait analysis. *Archives of Physical Therapy Medicine and Rehabilitation*, 65, 517-521.

In: Electromyography
Editor: Hiroki Takada

ISBN: 978-1- 62081-717-9

Chapter VI

Facial Electromyography as a Measure of Effort during Physical and Mental Tasks

Helma M. de Morree[1,2] and Samuele M. Marcora[3]
[1] School of Sport, Health and Exercise Sciences, Bangor University, United Kingdom
[2] Department of Medical Psychology and Neuropsychology, Center of Research on Psychology in Somatic diseases (CoRPS), Tilburg University, The Netherlands
[3] Centre for Sports Studies, University of Kent at Medway, United Kingdom

Abstract

Facial electromyography (EMG) is a psychophysiological technique that is often used in the study of emotions. However, there is also some research employing this technique to study the facial expression of effort. Using facial EMG, it has been shown that facial muscle activity is related to effort during mental tasks. It was found that facial EMG amplitude increases with task difficulty and with time on task during a two-choice serial reaction task. However, a relationship between facial EMG and effort has not always been found during mental tasks.

Recently, we have started to employ facial EMG to study effort during physical tasks. We have found, by manipulating exercise intensity and muscle fatigue during a leg-extension task, that facial EMG correlates positively with effort during weightlifting exercise. We have also demonstrated that facial EMG reflects exercise intensity during constant-workload cycling to exhaustion. Interestingly, we found that facial EMG increases significantly with exercise duration during high-intensity cycling, but not during moderate-intensity cycling.

A plausible neurobiological mechanism that might explain the relationship between facial EMG and effort is motor overflow. Motor overflow refers to involuntary muscle contractions that may accompany voluntary muscle contractions. This is thought to be caused by spreading of excitation in the motor cortex, because of increased excitability. In healthy adults, motor overflow is usually seen only during tasks that require considerable (physical) effort. This might explain the difference between high-intensity exercise, where the relationship between facial EMG and effort is strong and consistent, and moderate-intensity exercise or mental tasks, where a relationship between facial EMG and effort has not consistently been found.

Facial EMG may be used in the future along side rating of perceived effort as an extra, more objective measure of effort. This might have additional value in groups of people who have difficulties with rating effort, or when it is hard to obtain ratings, for example during maximal efforts of a few seconds and very high-intensity exercise of short duration. An additional benefit of facial EMG as a measure of effort is that it is a continuous measure.

Introduction

Facial electromyography (EMG) is a psychophysiological measure that is commonly used to measure facial muscle activity, for example in the study of emotion (Larsen, Berntson, Poehlmann, Ito, & Cacioppo, 2008). Two important facial muscles that have often been investigated are the zygomaticus major and the corrugator supercilii. These muscles are respectively important in smiling and frowning, and have been studied in relation to positive and negative affect (Larsen, Norris, & Cacioppo, 2003). The zygomaticus major pulls the lip corners up and back, and the corrugator supercilii draws the brows together and inward, producing vertical furrows between the brows (Tassinary, Cacioppo, & Vanman, 2007). Other facial muscles that are regularly studied are the frontalis, which raises the brows and thereby produces horizontal furrows in the forehead, the orbicularis oculi, which tightens the skin around the eyes, the procerus and the depressor supercilii, which pull the medial part of the brows downward and wrinkle the skin over the bridge of the nose, the levator labii, which raises the centre of the upper lip and flares the nostrils, the depressor anguli oris, which pulls the lip corners downward, and the orbicularis oris, which tightens, compresses, protrudes, and/or inverts the lips (Tassinary et al., 2007).

There are good reviews about the use of facial EMG in the study of emotions (e.g. Larsen et al., 2008). However, to the best of our knowledge, this chapter is the first to provide an overview of research on the facial expression of effort. Possibly the first to describe the facial expression of effort was Charles Darwin. In his book *The Expression of the Emotions in Man and Animals* (1872) he stated about frowning that it expresses "the perception of something difficult or disagreeable, either in thought or action" (p. 225). A few decades later, Robert Tait McKenzie described the face of effort in more detail. Included in an article by McKenzie in the Journal of Anatomy and Physiology (1905) is a photograph of a clay mask sculptured by the author himself, which clearly displays the facial expression of effort (see Figure 1). McKenzie describes the facial expression of effort as follows: "The face ... will show a general converging of the lines to the root of the nose, with transverse wrinkles over the bridge. The frowning brows are drawn down and the eye is narrowed to a mere slit. The outer angle of the eye shows the *crow's feet* accompanying all violent action of the muscles that close it." (McKenzie, 1924, pp. 19-20). Ever since these first observations, the facial expression of effort has received little attention in the scientific literature, even though it is very intuitive that frowning is linked to effort.

The feeling of effort is thought to have several important functions; it provides information about task difficulty, it limits energy consuming behaviour, and it contributes to the sense of agency (Preston & Wegner, 2009). The facial expression of effort presumably extends the functional importance of this sensation by revealing to others the effort exerted by an individual. Indeed, it has been demonstrated that people can judge the effort exerted by an athlete from non-verbal behaviours, including grimacing and squinting (Rejeski & Lowe, 1980). We therefore think that it is important to revive the study of the facial expression of effort.

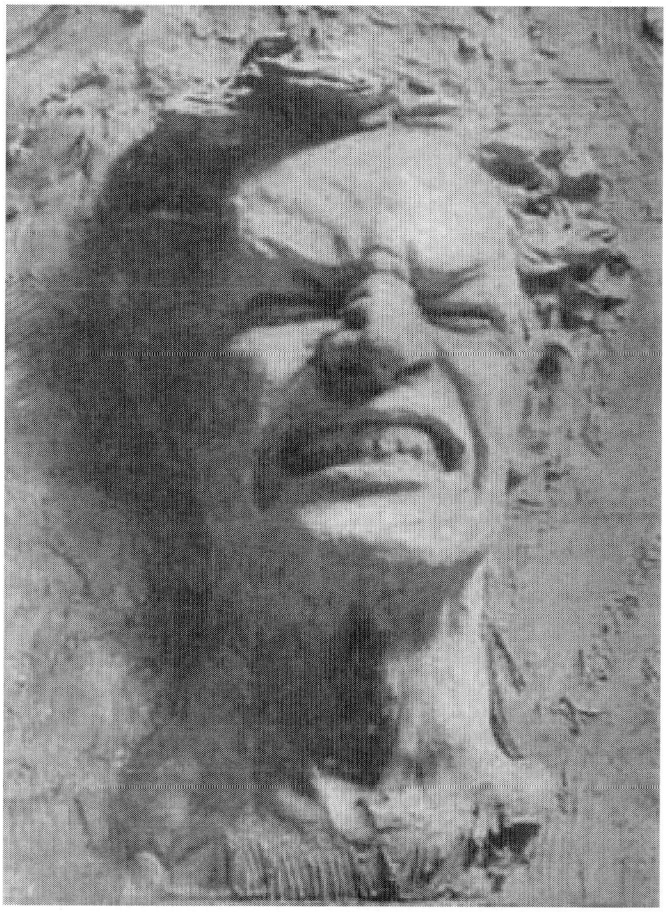

Figure 1. Photograph of a clay mask displaying the typical face of effort. The mask was sculptured by Robert Tait McKenzie from a snapshot of B.J. Wefers, a celebrated sprinter. Reprinted from Journal of Anatomy and Physiology, 40, R. Tait McKenzie, The facial expression of violent effort, breathlessness, and fatigue, 51-56, Copyright (1905), with permission from Wiley-Blackwell.

Facial Electromyography and Effort during Mental Tasks

The results of early studies on facial EMG suggested that activity of the corrugator supercilii and other facial muscles reflects effort during mental tasks (Cacioppo, Petty, & Morris, 1985; Smith, 1989). A few studies have since examined the relationship between facial EMG and task difficulty or effort during various mental tasks. Van Boxtel & Jessurun (1993) demonstrated that EMG activity of the frontalis, corrugator supercilii, and orbicularis oris inferior muscles increases with task difficulty during a two-choice serial reaction task. Task difficulty was manipulated by varying the stimulus presentation rate and hence also the required response rate.

Using a serial response task again, Waterink and van Boxtel (1994) have shown that EMG activity of these facial muscles increases over time as well. This was true whether stimulus presentation rate was self-paced or externally paced, but only occurred for participants whose performance remained stable during the course of the task. For participants whose performance declined during the task, the facial EMG activity also demonstrated a decreasing trend toward the end of the task. The authors suggested that these results support the notion that facial EMG activation reflects investment of effort in tasks that require sustained attention.

These results suggest that facial EMG indeed correlates with effort during mental tasks. However, effort ratings associated with these serial response tasks were not measured, and therefore no correlation could be calculated between facial EMG amplitude and perceived effort.

Other authors have not found a relationship between facial EMG and effort during mental tasks. Capa, Audiffren, & Ragot (2008a) found no effect of task difficulty on corrugator EMG during a visual memory search task with three levels of difficulty, even though significant effects of task difficulty were found on perceived difficulty and perceived level of mental effort.

The authors note that the most difficult condition was rated as moderately difficult while the easier two conditions were rated as relatively easy. Similarly, Silvestrini & Gendolla (2009) investigated the effects of task difficulty on corrugator EMG during memory tasks, and they did not find a difference in facial EMG between an easy memory task (memorising and recalling a list of 4 letter series) and a difficult memory task (memorising and recalling a list of 8 letter series), even though they found increased subjective difficulty ratings in the difficult task compared to the easy task. Judging from the reported means, the more difficult condition was rated as moderately difficult. In another study by Capa, Audiffren & Ragot (2008b), task difficulty was manipulated by varying the compatibility of the stimulus-response mapping.

The incompatible mapping condition was perceived to be more difficult than the compatible mapping condition, but facial EMG activation did not vary across these conditions. However, difficulty of goal instruction was also varied. One goal condition (react as quickly as possible without making errors) was perceived to be less difficult than a second goal condition (improve reaction times compared to a reference score without increasing error rates). Facial EMG activity was greater in the difficult compared to the easy goal condition for the frontalis, corrugator supercilii, and orbicularis oris inferior muscles. For both types of difficulty condition, stimulus-response compatibility and goal instruction, the more difficult condition was rated close to the midpoint on the scale between very easy and very difficult.

There are many differences in design across these studies, and it is not yet clear why facial EMG activity reflects task difficulty for some of these mental tasks and not others. The level of perceived task difficulty is relatively moderate in these studies; results would perhaps be more consistent across studies if higher task difficulty levels were employed. It does seem to be the case that task difficulty involving increased speed of response or increased time on task are likely factors to be reflected in facial EMG. This may implicate motor demands as a factor influencing effort related facial EMG in mental tasks.

Facial Electromyography and Effort during Physical Tasks

Preliminary Evidence

Prior to our studies, facial EMG had never been measured during physical tasks for the purpose of quantifying effort. We therefore review some studies that provide clues about this relationship, even though their methods and purposes are different. One study involved filming the facial expression during prolonged muscle contractions, and it was found that the facial expression changed from an ordinary expression to a frowning one (Tanii, Sadoyama, Sanjo, & Kogi, 1973). Other studies have measured facial EMG during exercise. Graham and colleagues have recorded frontalis EMG activity during several physical tasks (Graham et al., 1986) to study the effectiveness of using this muscle for biofeedback. They found that frontalis EMG was increased above baseline during a sustained push-up task and a sustained leg-lifting task. They also found differences in frontalis activity between different exercise intensities for an arm task and a head/neck task, but not for a leg task. A study on corrugator responses to affective picture viewing during physical activity compared baseline corrugator activity during rest with baseline corrugator activity during cycling at very low (14% peak power output) and low (40% peak power output) exercise intensities (Smith & O'Connor, 2003). It was found that corrugator EMG amplitude increased significantly with exercise intensity. The authors also investigated the orbicularis oculi muscle activity, but they did not find an effect of exercise on the EMG of this muscle.

Facial Electromyography and Effort during Leg-Extension Exercise

We are the first to have investigated the relationship between facial EMG and perception of effort during physical exercise (de Morree & Marcora, 2010). Our first experiment was aimed at quantifying the facial expression of effort with facial EMG of the corrugator supercilii muscles, and at correlating this with ratings of perceived effort (RPE). We investigated the effects of two experimental manipulations, exercise intensity and muscle fatigue, during weightlifting exercise on a leg-extension bench. Twenty recreationally active male volunteers (aged 22 ± 2 years) took part in this experiment. First of all, we asked our participants to lift and hold four weights (20, 40, 60, and 80% of their one-repetition maximum (1RM)), three times each, for 3 s, separated by 2-min rest periods. Secondly, we randomly allocated the participants to either the fatigue group or the control group, to investigate the effects of muscle fatigue on facial EMG and perception of effort during lifting of the same absolute weights. The participants came in for the post-test after a minimum of 48 h. The fatigue group repeated the leg-extension protocol immediately after performing an eccentric fatiguing protocol developed by Skurvydas, Jascaninas, & Zachovajevas (2000). This protocol consists of 100 drop jumps from a 40 cm high platform and is known to induce a significant strength loss (Marcora, Bosio, & de Morree, 2008; Nielsen, Madsen, Jorgensen, & Sahlin, 2005; Skurvydas, Dudoniene, Kalvenas, & Zuoza, 2002). Indeed, the protocol induced an average strength loss (measured by maximal voluntary contraction (MVC) before and after the fatiguing protocol) in the leg-extensor muscles of 23%. The control group repeated just the leg-extension protocol.

Throughout the protocol, muscle activity of the corrugator supercilii was measured with bipolar, single differential surface EMG (facial EMG). On both sides of the face, one electrode was placed immediately lateral to the glabellar midline and the other lateral to it, just above the medial edge of the eyebrow (Tassinary, Cacioppo, & Geen, 1989). Participants rated their effort directly after each lift on a modified CR10 scale for RPE (Borg, 1998).

This scale ranges from 0 (*no effort at all*) to 10 (*"maximal" effort*), and includes standard verbal anchors of perception of effort, such as *light*, *moderate*, and *hard (heavy)*, for intermediate values. In the instructions, we emphasised that the rating should be based exclusively on effort and not on any burning sensation (pain) in the legs. We defined effort to the participants as how hard they had to drive their leg to lift the weight (Hamilton, Killian, Summers, & Jones, 1996). In addition, we measured bipolar single differential surface EMG of the vastus lateralis muscle (leg EMG) during all lifts. For facial EMG and leg EMG we calculated the root mean square (RMS) for each lift during a 2 s plateau, detected from the data of a goniometer placed on the knee. The average of the three lifts at each intensity was used for statistical analysis.

Unless otherwise noted, data are presented as means ± standard deviations. RPE and leg EMG data were analysed using a three-way mixed ANOVA with test (pre vs. post) and exercise intensity (20, 40, 60, and 80% 1RM) as within-subjects factors, and group (fatigue vs. control) as the between-subjects factor. We tested for a significant test x group interaction and a main effect of exercise intensity. Facial EMG data were analysed using a four-way mixed ANOVA with an extra within-subjects factor recording site (left vs. right). We tested for a significant test x group interaction, a main effect of exercise intensity, and a main effect of electrode site. The within-subjects correlation coefficient (*r*) was calculated between RPE and facial EMG (average of left and right) for both tests and both groups separately using the method described by Bland & Altman (1995). Significance was set at 0.05 (two-tailed) for all analyses, which were conducted using the Statistical Package for the Social Sciences version 14 (SPSS Inc., Chicago, IL).

The results of this experiment are presented in Figure 2. The weights that participants had to lift during both the pre-test and the post-test, were 11 ± 2, 22 ± 4, 33 ± 6, and 44 ± 8 kg. RPE and leg EMG amplitude increased significantly with exercise intensity (main effects of exercise intensity: RPE, $p < 0.001$; leg EMG, $p < 0.001$). Facial EMG amplitude also increased significantly with exercise intensity (main effect of exercise intensity: $p < 0.001$). There was no significant difference between left and right electrode sites (main effect of electrode site: $p = 0.926$). Figure 2 therefore shows the average of both sites.

After the eccentric fatiguing protocol, RPE and leg EMG amplitude were significantly increased in the fatigue group, despite the fact that participants were lifting the same weights, but there was no difference between pre-test and post-test in the control group (test x group interactions: RPE, $p = 0.001$; leg EMG, $p = 0.025$). Facial EMG amplitude was also significantly increased during muscle fatigue in the fatigue group, with no change from pre-test to post-test in the control group (test x group interaction, $p = 0.029$). We found significant correlations between RPE and facial EMG for both conditions and both groups ($r = 0.61$-0.71, $p < 0.01$).

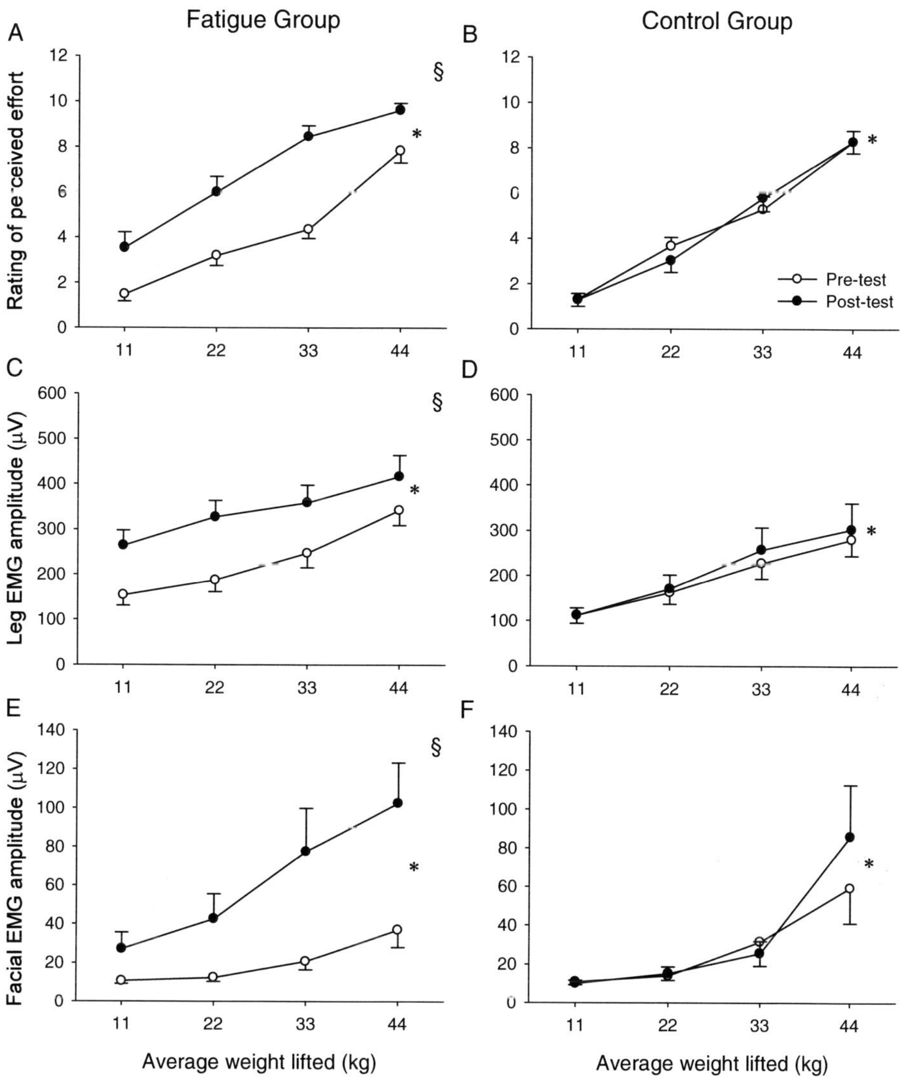

Figure 2. Effects of exercise intensity and muscle fatigue on rating of perceived effort, leg EMG (electromyogram), and facial EMG (average of left and right recording sites) during leg-extension exercise. * Significant main effect of exercise intensity ($p < 0.05$). § Significant test x group interaction ($p < 0.05$). Data are presented as means ± standard errors. Reprinted from Biological Psychology, 85, H.M. de Morree & S.M. Marcora, The face of effort: frowning muscle activity reflects effort during a physical task, 377-382, Copyright (2010), with permission from Elsevier.

Facial Electromyography and Effort during Cycling Exercise

Our second experiment (de Morree & Marcora, 2012) was aimed at corroborating and extending our findings to aerobic exercise. We therefore investigated the effects of exercise intensity and exercise duration on facial EMG and RPE during constant-workload cycling to exhaustion. Twenty recreationally active male and female volunteers (aged 25 ± 4 years) took part in this experiment. The test started with a 3-min warm-up at 30% of peak power output (P_{peak}), and this was followed by a rectangular workload until exhaustion. Participants were randomly allocated to either the high-intensity (power output at respiratory compensation point (P_{RCP})) or the moderate-intensity (P_{RCP} −20%) group. We asked them to cycle within ± 5 rpm of their preferred pedalling rate, which we had established during the preliminary session. Time to exhaustion (TTE) was measured from the start of the rectangular workload until the cadence dropped > 5 rpm below the required pedalling rate for > 5 s. The average workload during the TTE test was 63 ± 3% P_{peak} (219 ± 41 W) for the moderate-intensity group, and 80 ± 5% P_{peak} (284 ± 45 W) for the high-intensity group.

Throughout the TTE test, bipolar, single differential surface EMG was recorded from the bilateral corrugator supercilii muscles (facial EMG). On both sides of the face, one electrode was placed immediately lateral to the glabellar midline and the other lateral to it, just above the medial edge of the eyebrow (Tassinary et al., 1989). From the facial EMG data, we calculated the RMS over 1-min periods. Participants rated their effort during the final 15 s of each minute on a CR10 scale for RPE (Borg, 1998), which was displayed throughout the test. This scale ranges from 0 (*no effort at all*) to 10 (*"maximal" effort*), and includes standard verbal anchors of perception of effort, such as *light*, *moderate*, and *hard (heavy)*, for intermediate values. We defined effort to the participants as how hard they had to drive their legs (Hamilton et al., 1996) and how heavy their breathing was. We emphasised that the rating should be based exclusively on the effort it would take to pedal and to breathe and not on any pain in the legs. Heart rate was measured throughout the cycling test with a telemetric heart rate monitor.

Because of the different durations of the TTE test for the two intensities, we could directly compare the RPE, heart rate, and facial EMG data only for the first 5 min of the TTE test. However, in this chapter we also present previously unpublished data for the rest of the TTE test on a time-scale relative to TTE. RPE, heart rate (1-min averages), and facial EMG (average of left and right) data were analysed using two-way mixed ANOVAs with within-subjects factor exercise duration (1-5 min, and 0 [first min of rectangular workload], 25, 50, 75, and 100% [last min before exhaustion] of TTE), and between-subjects factor exercise intensity (moderate vs. high). Significant duration x intensity interactions were followed-up by one-way repeated measures ANOVAs with factor exercise duration for the two intensities separately, and we tested for simple main effects of exercise intensity at the different time points by using Holm-Bonferroni corrected (Holm, 1979) independent *t* tests. Differences between means were analysed with independent *t* tests also in case of other between-subjects differences, and with paired *t* tests in case of within-subjects differences. Significance was set at 0.05 (two-tailed) for all analyses, which were conducted using the Statistical Package for the Social Sciences version 14 (SPSS Inc., Chicago, IL).

The results of this experiment are presented in Figures 3 and 4. TTE was significantly different between the moderate-intensity and high-intensity groups (moderate: 25.8 ± 9.5 min, high: 6.8 ± 2.0 min; $p < 0.001$). For the first 5 min of the TTE test (Figure 3), RPE increased significantly over time (main effect of exercise duration: $p < 0.001$), and it was significantly higher for the high-intensity group compared to the moderate-intensity group (main effect of exercise intensity: $p = 0.002$). Follow-up of the significant duration x intensity interaction ($p < 0.001$) revealed that RPE increased significantly with exercise duration in both the moderate- and the high-intensity group (moderate, $p < 0.001$; high, $p < 0.001$). RPE was higher in the high-intensity group than in the moderate-intensity group at all time points (simple main effects of exercise intensity: $p \leq 0.021$), except for minute 1. Heart rate also increased significantly over time (main effect of exercise duration: $p < 0.001$), but the difference between the two intensities did not reach significance (main effect of exercise intensity: $p = 0.089$). Follow-up of the significant duration x intensity interaction ($p = 0.022$) revealed that heart rate increased significantly with exercise duration in both the moderate- and the high-intensity group (moderate, $p < 0.001$; high, $p < 0.001$). Heart rate was significantly higher in the high-intensity group than in the moderate-intensity group only at minute 5 (simple main effect of exercise intensity: $p = 0.007$). We found that facial EMG increased significantly over time (main effect of exercise duration: $p = 0.009$), and it was higher in the high-intensity group compared to the moderate-intensity group (main effect of exercise intensity: $p = 0.014$).

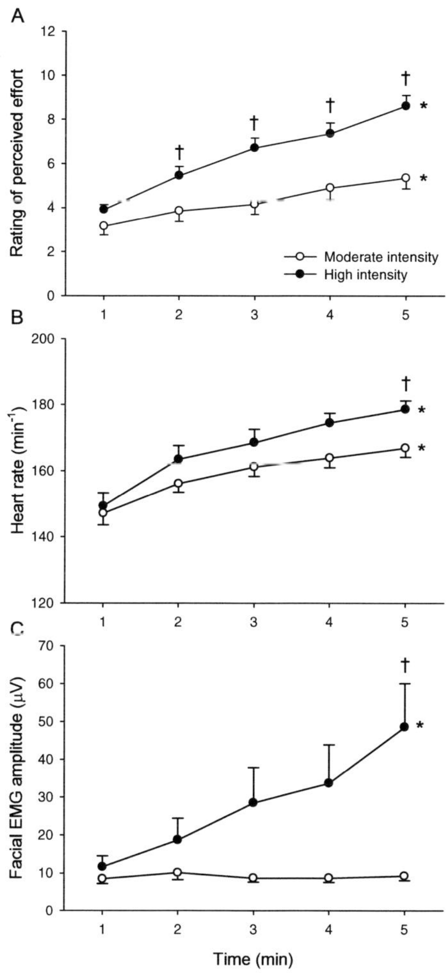

Figure 3. Effects of exercise duration and exercise intensity on rating of perceived effort, heart rate, and facial EMG (electromyogram) during the first 5 min of constant-workload cycling to exhaustion. In case of a significant duration x intensity interaction, only symbols for simple main effects are shown. * Significant simple main effect of exercise duration. † Significant simple main effect of exercise intensity. For heart rate: moderate intensity n = 10, high intensity, n = 9. Data are presented as means ± standard errors.

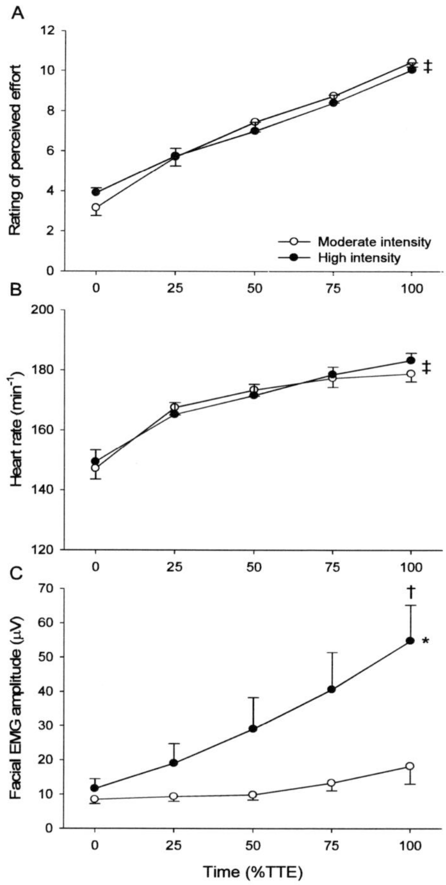

Figure 4. Effects of exercise duration and exercise intensity on rating of perceived effort, heart rate, and facial EMG (electromyogram) during constant-workload cycling to exhaustion. In case of a significant duration x intensity interaction, only symbols for simple main effects are shown. ‡ Significant main effect of exercise duration. * Significant simple main effect of exercise duration. † Significant simple main effect of exercise intensity. For heart rate: moderate intensity n = 10, high intensity n = 9. TTE = time to exhaustion. Data are presented as means ± standard errors.

Follow-up tests of the significant duration x intensity interaction ($p = 0.010$) revealed that facial EMG increased significantly with exercise duration in the high-intensity group ($p = 0.016$), but not in the moderate-intensity group ($p = 0.266$). Facial EMG was significantly higher in the high-intensity group than in the moderate-intensity group only at minute 5 (simple main effect of exercise intensity: $p = 0.003$).

For the data relative to TTE (Figure 4), RPE increased significantly over time (main effect of exercise duration: $p < 0.001$), but there was no significant difference between the two exercise intensities (main effect of exercise intensity: $p = 0.856$). There was also no significant difference in the increase over time between the two intensities (duration x intensity interaction: $p = 0.139$). The same pattern of results was found for heart rate (main effect of exercise duration: $p < 0.001$; main effect of exercise intensity: $p = 0.845$; duration x intensity interaction: $p = 0.229$). We found that facial EMG increased significantly over time (main effect of exercise duration: $p < 0.001$), and it was significantly higher in the high-intensity group than in the moderate-intensity group (main effect of exercise intensity: $p =$

0.012). Follow-up tests of the duration x intensity interaction ($p = 0.018$) revealed that facial EMG increased significantly with exercise duration in the high-intensity group ($p = 0.003$), but there was only a trend for an effect of exercise duration in the moderate-intensity group ($p = 0.071$). Facial EMG was significantly higher in the high-intensity group compared to the moderate-intensity group at 100% TTE (simple main effect of exercise intensity: $p = 0.006$).

Facial Electromyography and Effort during Sustained Leg-Extension Exercise

Our first experiment included a time to exhaustion test during which participants were required to sustain a leg extension with a weight equal to 20% 1RM, until they were not able to keep their leg in the extended position any longer (de Morree & Marcora, 2010, unpublished results). The pre-test data of ten participants of the leg-extension experiment (de Morree & Marcora, 2010) are included in this analysis. We measured facial EMG of the corrugator supercilii throughout this test, and we asked our participants to give their RPE every 30 s. Methods were as described above. TTE was 4.6 ± 1.0 min. Data were analysed at 0% (first 30 s), 25%, 50%, 75%, and 100% (last 30 s) of TTE. For facial EMG we calculated RMS values over 30-s periods. Not only did we investigate the effects of exercise duration during leg-extension exercise on RPE and facial EMG, we also compared the results with the RPE and facial EMG data relative to TTE from the cycling experiment (de Morree & Marcora, 2012, unpublished results).

RPE and facial EMG (average of left and right recording sites) data were initially analysed for the leg-extension exercise with one-way repeated measures ANOVAs with within-subjects factor exercise duration (0, 25, 50, 75, and 100% of TTE). RPE and facial EMG data were also analysed using a two-way mixed ANOVA with within-subjects factor exercise duration (0, 25, 50, 75, and 100% of TTE), and between-subjects factor exercise mode (moderate-intensity cycling, high-intensity cycling, and sustained leg extension). Post hoc pairwise comparisons were performed following Tukey's honestly significant difference procedure to correct for multiple comparisons. Significance was set at 0.05 (two-tailed) for all analyses, which were conducted using the Statistical Package for the Social Sciences version 16 (SPSS Inc., Chicago, IL).

The results are presented in Figure 5. RPE and facial EMG increased significantly over time during the sustained leg extension (main effect of exercise duration: RPE, $p < 0.001$; facial EMG, $p = 0.022$). When the sustained leg extension was compared to the cycling task, we did not find any differences in RPE, or in the increase in RPE over time (main effect of exercise duration: $p < 0.001$; main effect of exercise mode: $p = 0.332$; duration x mode interaction: $p = 0.120$). However, facial EMG was not the same in all exercise modes (main effect of exercise mode: $p = 0.026$; main effect of exercise duration: $p < 0.001$; duration x mode interaction: $p = 0.099$). Facial EMG was significantly higher in the high-intensity cycling than in the moderate-intensity cycling (pairwise comparison: $p = 0.032$), there was a trend for it to be higher during the sustained leg extension than during the moderate-intensity cycling (pairwise comparison: $p = 0.074$), and there was no significant difference between the sustained leg extension and the high-intensity cycling (pairwise comparison: $p = 0.922$).

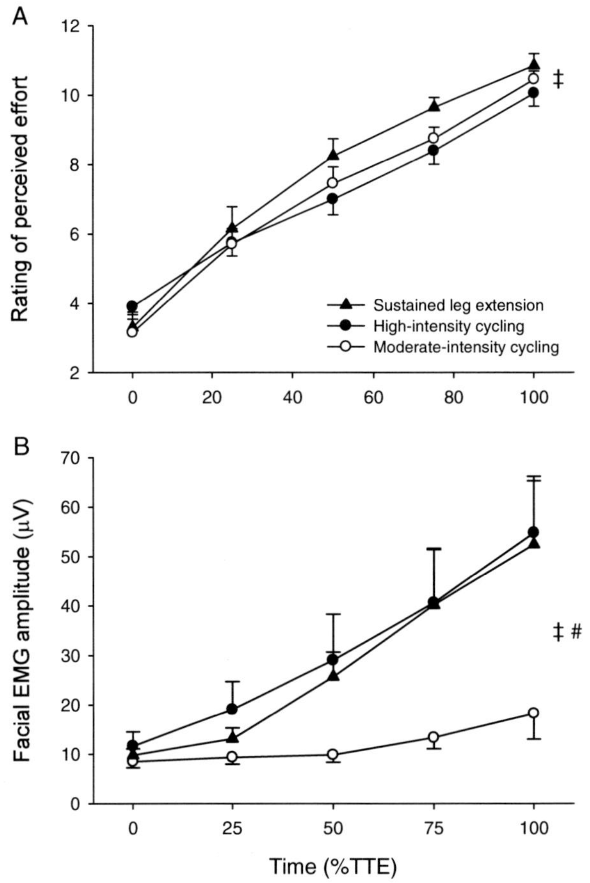

Figure 5. Effects of exercise duration and exercise mode on rating of perceived effort and facial EMG (electromyogram). # Significant main effect of exercise mode ($p < 0.05$). ‡ Significant main effect of exercise duration ($p < 0.05$). TTE = time to exhaustion. Data are presented as means ± standard errors.

Does Frowning Muscle Activity Reflect Perception of Effort?

The literature on the relationship between facial EMG and effort during mental tasks is ambivalent. Some studies have found that facial EMG reflects effort during mental tasks (van Boxtel & Jessurun, 1993; Waterink & van Boxtel, 1994), and others have not (always) found this relationship (Capa et al., 2008a; Capa et al., 2008b; Silvestrini & Gendolla, 2009). We were the first to measure facial EMG and perception of effort during physical tasks. During dynamic leg extensions, facial EMG amplitude correlated positively with perception of effort. Not only did facial EMG increase concomitantly with perception of effort when exercise intensity was increased, it was also increased concomitantly with an increase in perception of effort for the same exercise intensity when the leg-extensor muscles were weakened by muscle fatigue. Moreover, during a leg-holding task until exhaustion, we found that facial EMG and perception of effort both increased significantly over time. This result was very similar to the increase over time that we found in these two variables during high-intensity cycling to exhaustion. When we compared facial EMG and perception of effort during high-intensity and moderate-intensity constant-workload cycling to exhaustion, we found that, during the first 5 min of exercise, both variables were higher during high-intensity cycling compared to moderate-intensity cycling. This is in agreement with our finding that facial EMG and perception of effort both increased with exercise intensity during leg-extension exercise. However, an unexpected finding was that over the entire duration of the time to exhaustion test facial EMG and perception of effort were dissociated during moderate-intensity cycling. Perception of effort increased significantly over time, whereas facial EMG did not.

Perception of effort is thought to arise from corollary discharges of the central motor command from the premotor and motor areas of the brain to the muscles (Marcora, 2009). The facial expression of effort might be related to central motor command as well. It has been shown that the facial motor nucleus, which innervates the facial musculature, receives projections from cortical motor and premotor areas including the anterior cingulate cortex (Morecraft, Stilwell-Morecraft, & Rossing, 2004; Shackman et al., 2011). The relationship between effort and facial EMG might be explained by motor overflow in one or more of these areas. Motor overflow refers to (remote) involuntary muscle contractions that may accompany voluntary muscle contractions (Hoy, Fitzgerald, Bradshaw, Armatas, & Georgiou-Karistianis, 2004). This is thought to be caused by spreading of excitation in the motor cortex, because of increased excitability (Gandevia, 2001). In healthy adults, motor overflow is usually seen only during tasks that require considerable (physical) effort (Hoy et al., 2004). Most studies about motor overflow have focused specifically on motor overflow to homologous muscles on the opposite side of the body, called mirror movements (Espay, 2010). Unfortunately, in healthy adults there is very little research on motor overflow to the facial muscles, or synkinesis (Espay, 2010; Gandevia, 2001). It has been shown that motor overflow (to the contralateral limb) increases with increases in force output during finger flexions (Armatas, Summers, & Bradshaw, 1996). Furthermore, motor overflow (again to the contralateral limb) has been shown to increase during submaximal fatiguing finger abductions (Post, Bayrak, Kernell, & Zijdewind, 2008). These studies suggest that motor overflow may be proportional to the central motor command to the active muscles. The fact that facial EMG and effort seem to be related mainly during intense exercise and conditions of muscle fatigue, and not so much during lower intensity exercise and mental tasks is consistent with evidence that (contralateral) motor overflow is particularly noticeable under conditions of high levels of physical effort, involving high levels of absolute force, or muscle fatigue (Arányi & Rösler, 2002; Zijdewind & Kernell, 2001).

Directions for Future Research

Future investigations are needed to clarify why facial EMG did not significantly increase during moderate-intensity cycling, and why the relationship between effort and facial EMG is sometimes not found during mental tasks. One possible explanation is that motor overflow to facial musculature consistently occurs only when there is high output from the primary motor cortex (e.g. high-intensity exercise). During tasks with low motor demands, such as moderate-intensity exercise or some mental tasks, changes in perception of effort may be related to neurocognitive processes that do not result in significant motor overflow. It would be interesting to investigate the effects of a purely cognitive manipulation on facial EMG during a subsequent task. For example, mental fatigue has been shown to increase perception of effort during subsequent exercise, without any physiological changes (Marcora, Staiano, & Manning, 2009). This might therefore be the perfect manipulation to further investigate the 'cognitive component' of effort and its effect on facial EMG. If mental fatigue does not affect facial EMG during subsequent exercise, this would confirm our hypothesis that the facial expression of effort merely reflects the 'motor component' of effort.

It has been shown that people use non-verbal behaviours, including grimacing and squinting, to judge the effort exerted by others (Rejeski & Lowe, 1980), and we have demonstrated that frowning muscle activity reflects effort in several kinds of exercise. It would be interesting to investigate further how athletes might use this information during competitions. For a start, it would be interesting to investigate if athletes are aware of the facial expression of effort of themselves and others, and if they consciously use this in strategic decisions. The facial expression of effort might also affect perception of effort and exercise performance more directly. On the one hand, it has been shown that facial muscle contractions may increase force production in arm and leg muscles (Cartwright-Smith (1979) in Buck, 1980; Ebben, Leigh, & Geiser, 2008), and frowning might therefore be ergogenic. However, on the other hand, based on theories of embodied cognition (Niedenthal, 2007), one might expect that frowning would increase feelings of effort through facial feedback (Larsen, Kasimatis, & Frey, 1992; Strack & Neumann, 2000), and it might therefore be more ergogenic to smile during exercise. Future investigations should investigate the effects of frowning and smiling manipulations on perception of effort and exercise performance.

Methodological Considerations

Methodological issues such as electrode placement, signal detection, and signal analysis for EMG in general (De Luca, 2006), and facial EMG specifically (Fridlund & Cacioppo, 1986; Tassinary et al., 2007) are described in detail elsewhere. However, in this chapter we would like to bring to the attention some of the methodological issues that arise when using facial EMG to measure effort, especially during physical exercise.

Despite the fact that facial EMG is an objective measure, it is important to realise that, being a psychophysiological measure, it can be affected by social context. One source of potential bias is experimental demand confound. By attaching electrodes to the participant's face, you may make them more aware of their facial expressions. If the hypothesis of the study can be easily discerned, this might lead to participants purposely acting in accordance with the research hypothesis. The audience effect is also a potential source of bias during facial EMG recordings, as it has been shown that the presence of observers can affect facial EMG activity (e.g. Chapman, 1974). Another social factor to be aware of is mimicry. Facial EMG has been shown to be affected when participants watch facial expressions of others (e.g. Dimberg, 1982).

Bias from these social factors can be minimised by slight adaptations to the participant instructions and the experimental set-up. For example, experimenters can provide their participants with plausible alternative explanations about the purpose of the experiment and the nature of the recording, to minimise experimental demand confounds. If this approach is used, participants will need to be fully debriefed about the true purpose of the experiment at the end of testing. Experimenters can position themselves behind the participant during the task to make the participant feel less observed and to prevent mimicry. Encouragement and feedback during the task, like exercise physiologists are used to provide during maximal exercise to ensure that their participant exerts maximal effort, should be kept to a minimum.

Physical exercise is likely to induce movement artefacts. Though most of these predominantly low frequency artefacts can be filtered out with a high-pass filter, it is always better to prevent artefacts than to filter them out afterwards. Cable movement artefacts can be reduced by loosely fixating the cables with, for example, a headband. In the case of electrodes on the upper part of the face, it is advisable to lead the cables upward over the head and, if possible, down the back. Transpiration is another issue that needs to be accounted for when recording facial EMG during physical exercise. Even when the laboratory is kept cool (≤ 20 °C), it is likely that participants will sweat during effortful physical exercise. To prevent that electrodes will detach because of transpiration, a headband can be used to keep transpiration from running down the forehead to the electrodes, and in addition, a fan can be used to cool the participant.

With surface EMG recordings of the facial muscles, there is a relatively large chance that cross-talk will occur, because the facial muscles are relatively small, and several muscles are overlapping. Cross-talk is the detection of signals originating from muscles adjacent to the muscle of interest (De Luca, 2006). This can be minimised by proper electrode placement (Tassinary et al., 2007), but it is important to keep in mind that surface EMG is not selective and that your facial EMG recording might therefore reflect activity from several muscles within the region of your muscle of interest. However, this is not a problem if the cross-talk originates from muscles that have comparable effects on facial expression to the muscle of interest. For example, it is highly likely that surface electrodes placed over the corrugator supercilii also pick up signals from the procerus and the depressor supercilii (Fridlund & Cacioppo, 1986), and to a lesser extent from the orbicularis oculi and the frontalis. These muscles could all contribute to the facial expression of effort, and therefore cross-talk from these muscles does not affect our conclusions.

Practical Applications

Now that we have shown that facial EMG reflects perception of effort during several types of exercise, it could be used (during those types of exercise) along side rating of perceived effort as an extra, more objective measure of effort, taking into account the methodological issues discussed above. This might have additional value in groups of people who are incapable to rate effort because they have difficulties with self-monitoring, such as people with brain function disorders or children. Facial EMG might also be used when it is hard to obtain effort ratings due to the experimental design, for example during maximal efforts of a few seconds and very high-intensity exercise of short duration (≤ 2 min). An additional benefit of facial EMG as a measure of effort is that it is a continuous measure. Facial EMG could also be useful in situations where experimenters do not want to explicitly ask participants to attend to their perception of effort.

Conclusion

The literature shows that the relationship between facial EMG and effort during mental tasks is inconsistent. It is therefore necessary to further investigate which task characteristics determine facial expression during mental tasks. We have shown that facial EMG of the frowning muscles, possibly through motor overflow, reflects perception of effort during intense exercise, but not during lower-intensity exercise. More research is needed in the future to reveal why facial EMG reflects perception of effort in most, but not all, types of physical exercise.

References

Arányi, Z. & Rösler, K.M. (2002). Effort-induced mirror movements. A study of transcallosal inhibition in humans. *Experimental Brain Research*, 145, 76-82.

Armatas, C. A., Summers, J. J. & Bradshaw, J. L. (1996). Strength as a factor influencing mirror movements. *Human Movement Science*, 15, 689-705.

Bland, J. M. & Altman, D. G. (1995). Calculating correlation coefficients with repeated observations. Part 1 - Correlation within subjects. *British Medical Journal*, 310, 446.

Borg, G. A. (1998). *Borg's perceived exertion and pain scales*. Champaign, IL: Human Kinetics.

Buck, R. (1980). Nonverbal behavior and the theory of emotion: the facial feedback hypothesis. *Journal of Personality and Social Psychology*, 38, 811-824.

Cacioppo, J. T., Petty, R. E. & Morris, K. J. (1985). Semantic, evaluative, and self-referent processing: memory, cognitive effort, and somatovisceral activity. *Psychophysiology*, 22, 371-384.

Capa, R. L., Audiffren, M. & Ragot, S. (2008a). The interactive effect of achievement motivation and task difficulty on mental effort. *International Journal of Psychophysiology*, 70, 144-150.

Capa, R. L., Audiffren, M. & Ragot, S. (2008b). The effects of achievement motivation, task difficulty, and goal difficulty on physiological, behavioral, and subjective effort. *Psychophysiology*, 45, 859-868.

Chapman, A. J. (1974). An electromyographic study of social facilitation: a test of the 'mere presence' hypothesis. *British Journal of Psychology*, 65, 123-128.

Darwin, C. (1872). *The Expression of the emotions in man and animals*. London: John Murray Albemarle Street.

De Luca, C. (2006). Electromyography. In J. Webster (Ed.), *Encyclopedia of medical devices and instrumentation* (pp. 98-109). Hoboken, NJ: Wiley.

de Morree, H. M. & Marcora, S. M. (2010). The face of effort: frowning muscle activity reflects effort during a physical task. *Biological Psychology*, 85, 377-382.

de Morree, H. M. & Marcora, S. M. (2012). Frowning muscle activity and perception of effort during constant-workload cycling. *European Journal of Applied Physiology*,112, 1967-1972.

Dimberg, U. (1982). Facial reactions to facial expressions. *Psychophysiology*, 19, 643-647.

Ebben, W. P., Leigh, D. H. & Geiser, C. F. (2008). The effect of remote voluntary contractions on knee extensor torque. *Medicine and Science in Sports and Exercise*, 40, 1805-1809.

Espay, A. J. (2010). Motor excess during movement: Overflow, mirroring, and synkinesis. *Clinical Neurophysiology*, 121, 5-6.

Fridlund, A. J. & Cacioppo, J. T. (1986). Guidelines for human electromyographic research. *Psychophysiology*, 23, 567-589.

Gandevia, S. C. (2001). Spinal and supraspinal factors in human muscle fatigue. *Physiological Reviews*, 81, 1725-1789.

Graham, C., Cook, M. R., Cohen, H. D., Gerkovich, M. M., Phelps, J. W. & Fotopoulos, S. S. (1986). Effects of variation in physical effort on frontalis EMG activity. *Biofeedback and Self Regulation*, 11, 135-141.

Hamilton, A. L., Killian, K. J., Summers, E. & Jones, N. L. (1996). Quantification of intensity of sensations during muscular work by normal subjects. *Journal of Applied Physiology*, 81, 1156-1161.

Holm, S. (1979). A simple sequentially rejective multiple test procedure. *Scandinavian Journal of Statistics*, 6, 65-70.

Hoy, K. E., Fitzgerald, P. B., Bradshaw, J. L., Armatas, C. A. & Georgiou-Karistianis, N. (2004). Investigating the cortical origins of motor overflow. *Brain Research Reviews*, 46, 315-327.

Larsen, J. T., Norris, C. J. & Cacioppo, J. T. (2003). Effects of positive and negative affect on electromyographic activity over zygomaticus major and corrugator supercilii. *Psychophysiology*, 40, 776-785.

Larsen, J. T., Berntson, G. G., Poehlmann, K. M., Ito, T. A. & Cacioppo, J. T. (2008). The psychophysiology of emotion. In M. Lewis, J. M. Haviland-Jones, & L. Feldman Barrett (Eds.), *Handbook of Emotions* (3rd edition, pp. 180-195). New York: Guilford Press.

Larsen, R. J., Kasimatis, M. & Frey, K. (1992). Facilitating the furrowed brow: an unobtrusive test of the facial feedback hypothesis applied to unpleasant affect. *Cognition and Emotion*, 6, 321-338.

Marcora, S. (2009). Perception of effort during exercise is independent of afferent feedback from skeletal muscles, heart, and lungs. *Journal of Applied Physiology*, 106, 2060-2062.

Marcora, S. M., Bosio, A. & de Morree, H. M. (2008). Locomotor muscle fatigue increases cardiorespiratory responses and reduces performance during intense cycling exercise independently from metabolic stress. *American Journal of Physiology - Regulatory, Integrative and Comparative Physiology*, 294, R874-883.

Marcora, S. M., Staiano, W. & Manning, V. (2009). Mental fatigue impairs physical performance in humans. *Journal of Applied Physiology*, 106, 857-864.

McKenzie, R. T. (1905). The facial expression of violent effort, breathlessness, and fatigue. *Journal of Anatomy and Physiology*, 40, 51-56.

McKenzie, R. T. (1924). *Exercise in education and medicine* (3rd edition). Philadelphia: W. B. Saunders company.

Morecraft, R. J., Stilwell-Morecraft, K. S. & Rossing, W. R. (2004). The motor cortex and facial expression: new insights from neuroscience. *Neurologist*, 10, 235-249.

Niedenthal, P. M. (2007). Embodying emotion. *Science*, 316, 1002-1005.

Nielsen, J. S., Madsen, K., Jorgensen, L. V. & Sahlin, K. (2005). Effects of lengthening contraction on calcium kinetics and skeletal muscle contractility in humans. *Acta Physiologica Scandinavica*, 184, 203-214.

Post, M., Bayrak, S., Kernell, D. & Zijdewind, I. (2008). Contralateral muscle activity and fatigue in the human first dorsal interosseous muscle. *Journal of Applied Physiology*, 105, 70-82.

Preston, J. & Wegner, D. M. (2009). Elbow grease: when action feels like work. In E. Morsella, J. A. Bargh, & P. M. Gollwitzer (Eds.), *Oxford handbook of human action* (pp. 569-586). Oxford, United Kingdom: Oxford University Press.

Rejeski, W. J. & Lowe, C. A. (1980). Nonverbal expression of effort as causally relevant information. *Personality and Social Psychology Bulletin*, 6, 436-440.

Shackman, A. J., Salomons, T. V., Slagter, H. A., Fox, A. S., Winter, J. J. & Davidson, R. J. (2011). The integration of negative affect, pain and cognitive control in the cingulate cortex. *Nature Reviews Neuroscience*, 12, 154-167.

Silvestrini, N. & Gendolla, G. H. (2009). Mood-regulative hedonic incentive interacts with mood and task difficulty to determine effort-related cardiovascular response and facial EMG. *Biological Psychology*, 82, 54-63.

Skurvydas, A., Jascaninas, J. & Zachovajevas, P. (2000). Changes in height of jump, maximal voluntary contraction force and low-frequency fatigue after 100 intermittent or continuous jumps with maximal intensity. *Acta Physiologica Scandinavica*, 169, 55-62.

Skurvydas, A., Dudoniene, V., Kalvenas, A. & Zuoza, A. (2002). Skeletal muscle fatigue in long-distance runners, sprinters and untrained men after repeated drop jumps performed at maximal intensity. *Scandinavian Journal of Medicine and Science in Sports*, 12, 34-39.

Smith, C. A. (1989). Dimensions of appraisal and physiological response in emotion. *Journal of Personality and Social Psychology*, 56, 339-353.

Smith, J. C. & O'Connor, P. J. (2003). Physical activity does not disturb the measurement of startle and corrugator responses during affective picture viewing. *Biological Psychology*, 63, 293-310.

Strack, F. & Neumann, R. (2000). Furrowing the brow may undermine perceived fame: the role of facial feedback in judgements of celebrity. *Personality and Social Psychology Bulletin,* 26, 762-768.

Tanii, K., Sadoyama, T., Sanjo, Y. & Kogi, K. (1973). Appearance of effort-depending changes in static local fatigue. *Journal of Human Ergology*, 2, 31-45.

Tassinary, L. G., Cacioppo, J. T. & Geen, T. R. (1989). A psychometric study of surface electrode placements for facial electromyographic recording: I. The brow and cheek muscle regions. *Psychophysiology*, 26, 1-16.

Tassinary, L. G., Cacioppo, J. T. & Vanman, E. J. (2007). The skeletomotor system: surface electromyography. In J. T. Cacioppo, L. G. Tassinary, & G. G. Berntson (Eds.), *Handbook of psychophysiology* (3rd edition, pp. 267-299). Cambridge, United Kingdom: University Press.

van Boxtel, A. & Jessurun, M. (1993). Amplitude and bilateral coherency of facial and jaw-elevator EMG activity as an index of effort during a two-choice serial reaction task. *Psychophysiology*, 30, 589-604.

Waterink, W. & van Boxtel, A. (1994). Facial and jaw-elevator EMG activity in relation to changes in performance level during a sustained information processing task. *Biological Psychology*, 37, 183-198.

Zijdewind, I. & Kernell, D. (2001). Bilateral interactions during cntractions of intrinsic hand muscles. *Journal of Neurophysiology*, 85, 1907-1913.

Reviewed by Dr. Amy E. Hayes, Bangor University, United Kingdom.

In: Electromyography
Editor: Hiroki Takada

ISBN: 978-1- 62081-717-9

Chapter VII

Analysis of Facial Expressions for Mimetic Muscles by Using Electromyogram - Electromyogram Analysis of Facial Muscle During Tuning of Expression

Yasuhiro Ogoshi[1]*, Tomohiro Takezawa[2], Yoshinori Mitsuhashi[3], Sakiko Ogoshi[3], Hideaki Saito[1] and Chikahiro Araki[1]

[1]Graduate School of Engineering, University of Fukui, Fukui City, Japan
[2]Research and Education Program for Life Science,
University of Fukui, Eiheiji-cho, Japan
[3]Faculty of Education and Regional Studies,
University of Fukui, Research Postdoctoral Fellowship
of the Japan Society for the Promotion of Science (ISPS)
Fukui City, Japan,

Abstract

Facial expressions of human beings play an important role in understanding each other's feelings during communication. It has been reported that Japanese people have weaker facial expressions than Americans, i.e., Japanese people exhibit low levels of activity of mimetic muscles. This may be one of the reasons why it is more difficult to read facial expressions of Japanese people. In fact, it is difficult to analyze their facial expressions visually and by image processing.

It has been reported that when human beings feel a particular emotion, the facial muscles required for expressing that emotion show electromyogram (EMG) activity, even though the emotion was not expressed on their face. Thus, using Japanese male university

* E-mail: y-ogoshi@u-fukui.ac.jp.

students as subjects, EMG analysis was performed in this study to clarify how mimetic muscles work when Ekman's six facial expressions were expressed. To achieve a smoother and cooperative communication, humans read each other's emotions and behave sympathetically. One such behavior is called "tuning of expression" in which a person's expression is matched with that of his/her partner in a given conversation, either consciously or unconsciously. This behavior is difficult to confirm visually because the expression is often very weak; however, such facial muscle activities can be observed by means of EMG. In this study, university students were paired and each pair was asked to talk freely. Their facial muscle activities were observed while students consciously and unconsciously exhibited tuning of expression.

Keywords: Facial expression, Action units, Facial Action Coding System, Emotional contagion, Myo-Electric potential, Electromyograms

Introduction

Extensive studies of facial expressions have long been conducted in the fields of psychology and engineering. The research by Ekman et al. which lead to the Facial Action Coding System (FACS) (Ekman and Friesen, 1975; Ekman and Friesen, 1977) is well known. FACS has six expressions that are classified on the basis of six emotions: happy, surprised, sad, angry, disgusted, and fear.

Currently, many studies are conducted using this classification system. In FACS, facial structures called action units (AU) are separated into the smallest possible unit that can be perceived visually.

Furthermore, the movement of these units is defined in detail, and observations of the movement and relative positions of these AU can be applied to various forms of expression analyses. For example, there have been various applications such as visual analysis of video images of facial expressions by people, facial expression recognition through image processing, and simulation of facial expressions by means of computer graphics. When two human beings communicate with one another, one can experience the same emotion by perceiving the specific emotional expression of the other. "Emotional Contagion" (Doherty, 1997) is a measurement of this sensitivity to the emotional expression of others. The concept of emotional contagion evolved from a study of how the crying of an infant caused another infant to start crying (Hoffman, 1987). In addition, such phenomenon is not limited to a specific communication channel such as facial expression, but is carried out through various other communication channels such as speech and body movements. This paper limits the discussion to the communication channel of facial expressions. There appears to be a natural tendency to mirror observed expressions. This imitation of expression (Hatfield, Cacioppo and Rapson, 1992) is known to arise spontaneously and unintentionally. The "Impression Rating Method" is an attempt at a systemic identification of facial expression and allows an evaluator to judge the expression of the subject through observation. However, the visual assessment by the evaluator is far from being objective. Moreover, detecting small changes in facial expressions is difficult when analyzing by means of computer image processing.

Lundqvist revealed that an adult expresses the same facial expression as one's interactional partner and when one was shown photographs of stimulating facial expressions of others (Gump and Kulik, 1997; Tomkins, 1962; Tomkins, 1963), the observer's facial muscles showed electrical potential activity (Lundqvist, 1995). The study on facial muscles during the forming of facial expression (Sonnby–Börgstom, Jönsson and Svensson, 2003), examined the relationship between emotional empathy and imitation of facial expressions.

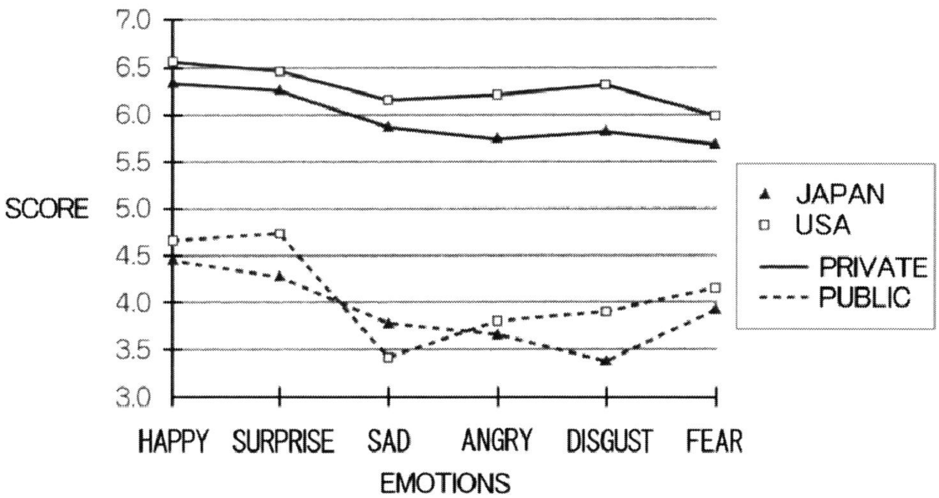

Figure 1. Emotional expressions of Americans and Japanese in public and private situations.

In this study, it was clarified that people with very high emotional empathy showed electrical potential activity of facial muscles similar to the facial expressions presented at an extremely short reaction time of 56 ms.

In contrast, people with low emotional empathy did not show this behavior. Sonnby–Börgstom et al. also examined emotional expressions related to gender differences (Sonnby–Börgstom, Jönsson and Svensson, 2008). Women were reported to present higher degrees of facial expression of happiness and disgust. On the other hand, while there was no gender difference for the facial expressions of sadness and happiness and men suppressed their facial responses to emotions more so than women.

Figure 1 shows the survey reports of emotional expressions of Americans and Japanese in public and private occasions (Nakamura, 1992). It shows six emotions and suggests that in general, emotional expressions of Japanese are less than that of Americans.

In this study, based on the reports from Lundqvist (Lundqvist, 1995) investigations were carried out on facial expressions of Japanese people, which are considered difficult to read visually, by employing electromyograms (EMG) of the activities of facial muscles. EMGs data was acquired from Japanese male university students while they expressed six emotions: happiness, surprise, sadness, anger, disgust, and fear.

In addition, observations were made concerning the tuning of facial expressions of students by pairing them and conducting a fun conversation while they face each other. EMG data was analyzed for cases when students carried out conscious and unconscious tuning of expression.

Method for Measuring for Facial Muscles Function with an Electromyogram

The Specifications and setup of the apparatus used in the EMG measurement of the facial muscles.

1) Electrodes

The specifications of electrodes used in our experiment are as follows:

- electrode material (Ag/AgCl), NIHON KOHDEN CORPORATION, Japan, NE-113A
- lectrode geometry (discs)
- size (7mm in diameter)
- use of gel or paste, alcohol applied to cleanse skin, skin abrasion
- interelectrode distance 13 mm apart

2) EMG Electrode Placements

The electrodes were affixed on the subjects as presented in Figure 2 accordance with "Guidelines for human Electromyographic Research" (Fridlund and Cacioppo, 1986).

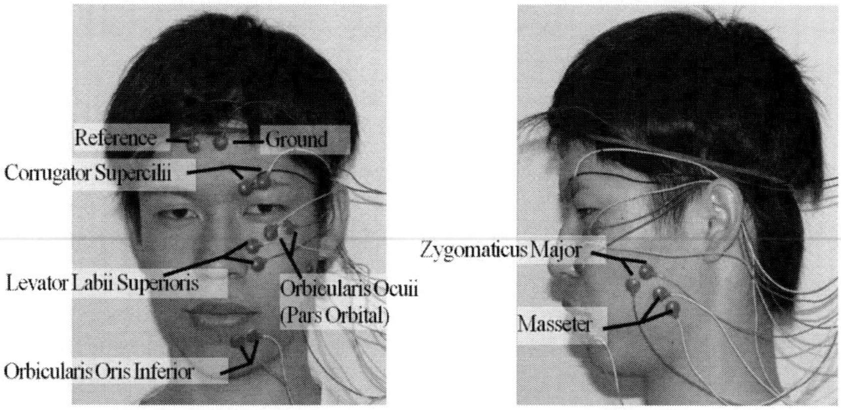

Figure 2. demonstrates the pasting position of the electrode.

The six facial muscles targeted for measurement in our experiment were as follows:

- Corrugator Supercilii
- Orbicularis Oculi
- Levator Labii Superioris
- Orbicularis Oris Inferior
- Zygomaticus Major
- Masseter

3) Sampling EMG into the Computer

The following combination Analog/Digital converter and Electroencephalographic Amplifier was used to obtain EMG measurements.

The model, resolving power, and sampling rate were as follows:

- Electroencephalographic Amplifier, DIGITEX LAB Co., Ltd. , Japan, Polymate AP1532
- Sampling rate 1000Hz
- AD -Card 32ch 16bits

4) Amplification

The specifications of the amplifier contained in the Electroencephalographic Amplifier profiled in 3) are as follows:

- differential
- input impeadance 10 MΩ
- Common Mode Rejection Ratio (CMRR) 86 dB or more
- actual gain range used from x100 to x1000

5) Filtering of the Raw EMG

The Electroencephalographic Amplifier outlined in 3) was set as follows:

- low and high pass filters
- filter types Butterworth
- low pass cut-off frequencies 10Hz and high pass cut-off frequencies 500Hz

6) EMG Processing

The signal gathered by the Electroencephalographic Amplifier shown in 3) was smoothed as follows:

- Smoothing with a low-pass filter with a time constant of 30 ms.

7) EMG Normalization

The signal processed above was normalized as follows:

- The EMG associated with 100% MVC (Maximal Voluntary Contraction) is designated as 100%.

8) How Subjects Were Trained to Obtain MVC

For the subjects to carry out the maximum voluntary contraction, sufficient preliminary training of each facial muscle was performed as follows:

- Corrugator Supercilii
- Strongly furrow the brow
- Orbicularis Oculi
- Strongly raise the cheeks and blink
- Levator Labii Superioris
- Strongly lift the nose and upper lip
- Orbicularis Oris Inferior
- Shut the mouth and strongly point forward
- Zygomaticus Major
- Strongly raise the corner of the mouth
- Masseter
- Perform the movement of biting hard

Experiment-1: EMG Measurements During the Six Expressions

1) Subjects

Six Japanese male university students were used as subjects with a mean age of 22.5 years.

2) Six Target Expressions

Expressions used in this experiment are Ekman's six expressions: happiness, surprise, sadness, anger, disgust, and fear, as well as an additional neutral expression we called expressionless. Figure 3 demonstrates these six expressions performed by a subject.

Furthermore, it is difficult to obtain accurate measurements since the interpretation and understanding of these expressions differ for each subject. Therefore, pictures of the six expressions (Ekman and Friesen, 1975) were presented to all subjects. These expressions are considered universal, i.e., common to all humans regardless of culture.

To gain an understanding from the subjects, the characteristic of the movement of each facial muscle necessary to create an expression was explained in detail. Then, the subjects were asked to perform these six expressions. Training in the formation of the expressions was conducted in which all subjects and many researchers participated. Training was repeated until everyone was able to present and distinguish the expressions. The pasting position of the electrodes (Figure 2), measuring equipment settings, and data processing were as previously outlined in this manuscript.

3) The EMG Measurement Method for the Six Expressions + Impassive

After the electrodes were affixed on the subjects, as outlined in figure 2, EMG was measured for the maximum voluntary contraction of each facial muscle. Next, as shown in Figure 4, subjects were asked to be expressionless for the first five seconds, then to express and preserve an expression for the next 10 s, and again to be expressionless for the last five seconds. As demonstrated in figure 4, EMG was measured for the six expressions (happiness, surprise, sadness, anger, disgust, fear) + expressionless.

4) EMG Measurement Results during the Six Expressions + Expressionless

For each facial muscle and each process (expression) shown in Figure 5, the mean amplitude was derived for the first five seconds when the subject remained expressionless and then for the ten seconds when their expressions changed. The differences in amplitudes were set as the mean response value. % MVC was calculated by using the average of the absolute value of EMG values obtained over a one second interval at a sampling rate of 1000Hz divided by the average of the absolute value of EMG values obtained over a one second interval at a sampling rate of 1000Hz while the average maximum voluntary contraction force was observed previously for each muscle during training.

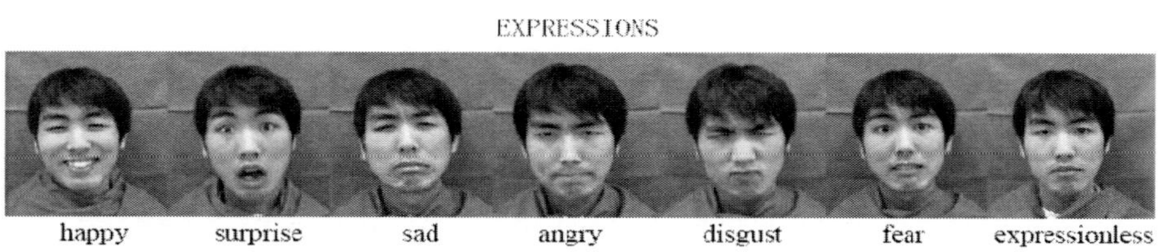

Figure 3. Six expressions performed by a subject.

These calculations were performed for each subject. Figure 5 demonstrates the standardized results obtained from all six subjects.

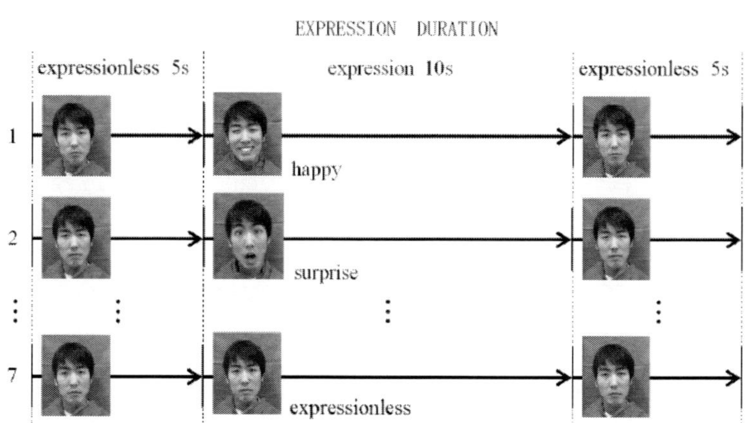

(EMG measurement for the six expressions + expressionless).

Figure 4. Flow of facial muscle measurement during exhibition of expressions.

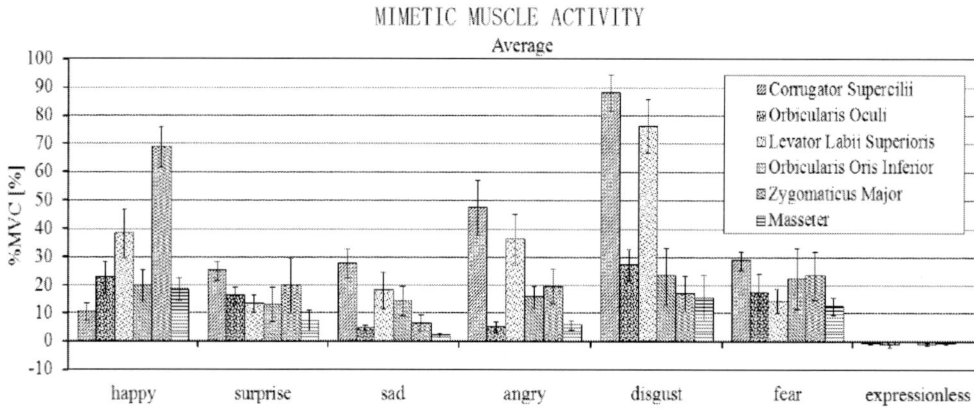

Figure 5. The state of activity of each mimetic muscle for each expression.

5) Examination of EMG during the Six Expressions + Expressionless

Here, the activity of each mimetic muscle is described according to the expression. For the facial expression of happiness, there were strong activities for Zygomaticus Major muscles. There were some activities in the other muscles with the except for the Corrugator Supercilii muscle which showed low activity.

At that time, the activity of the Zygomaticus Major muscle was found to be much stronger than that of other facial expressions. For the expression of anger, Corrugator Supercilii and Levator Labii Superioris brow muscles showed strong activities.

Activities in the Orbicularis Oris Inferior and Zygomaticus Major muscle were fairly strong, while activities in the Orbicularis Oculi and Masseter muscle were found to be weak.

For the expression of disgust, Corrugator Supercilii and Levator Labii Superioris muscle showed strong activities. In particular, these muscles were found to be highly active relative to other muscles. For the facial expression of sadness, some activities were observed in the Corrugator Supercilii, Orbicularis Oris Inferior and Levator Labii Superioris, but other mimetic muscles did not show much activity.

In addition, all mimetic muscle activities showed uniformity, and no special characteristics were observed. For the expression of disgust, Corrugator Supercilii and Levator Labii Superioris muscle showed strong activities.

In particular, these muscles were found to be highly active relative to other muscles. For the expression of surprise and fear, Corrugator Supercilii and Zygomaticus Major muscle showed relatively strong activities, but there was no particular activity in any of the mimetic muscles, and no special characteristics were observed.

In this experiment, similarities in characteristics were found in the formation of the expressions of surprise and fear. In addition, the Corrugator Supercilii muscle was found to be highly active in the formation of every facial expression, but it is thought that electric potential activities of other muscles around Corrugator Supercilii were mixed. Our EMG data concurs with and supports observations and descriptions of facial muscle activity put forth by Ekman (Ekman and Friesen, 1975).

Experiment-2: EMG Measurement during the Tuning of Expression

1) Subjects

The same six Japanese male university students were used as subjects in this experiment. They were asked to form pairs and the three pairs participated in the subsequent experiment.

2) EMG Measurement during Intentional Tuning of Expression

(1) Subjects were paired, with A being the subject performing the expression and B being the subject observing the expression. Both subjects A and B maintained the same electrodes attached to their face, as used in the EXPERIMENT-1. EXPERIMENT-2 was conducted following the completion of EXPERIMENT-1.
(2) As shown in Figure 6, two subjects and one instructor enter the laboratory. Subjects A and B sit on chairs facing each other. The instructor stands such that only subject A can see him/her; the instructor gives a signal to subject A to deliberately smile. In this study, the instructor presses a button to send a trigger signal to the EMG measurement device. Subject B receives the facial expression from subject A, and returns an intentional smile. This process is repeated three times.
(3) Next, the roles of subjects A and B are switched, and step (2) is performed again.
(4) Steps (2)–(3) were carried out on all three pairs.

Furthermore, pasting position of the electrodes on the face of subjects A and B, and settings of measurement instruments in EXPERIMENT-2 are the same as those in EXPERIMENT-1. Data processing in EXPERIMENT-2 differed from experiment in that %MVC was not calculated and raw EMG data was analysed.

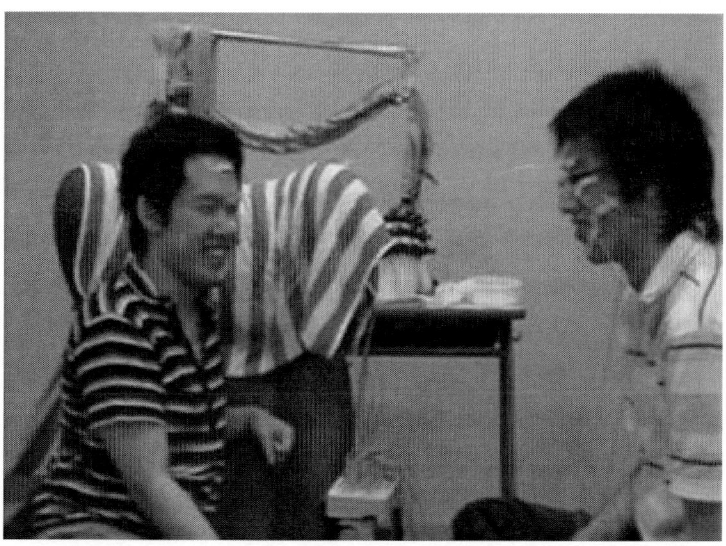

Figure 6. Situation in the laboratory during observations of the spontaneous and intentional tuning of expression.

3) EMG Measurement for the Tuning of Expression That Occurs Unconsciously

The following experiments are carried out using the same subjects who carried out the above experiment.

(1) The subjects formed pairs and were asked to choose a fun topic that might be common to university students (such as part-time work experiences, recently watched movies, themes of interests). The subjects talked freely for 5 min, without being preoccupied about their expressions and only concentrating on making the conversation enjoyable. They were to interact naturally, without intentionally performing expressions or choosing which subject was to present or observe expressions.
(2) The interactions were captured on video and EMG measurements were carried out.
(3) The steps (1)–(2) were performed on all three pairs.

Subsequently, the pair's electrical potential activity of the mimetic muscles during the tuning of expression was analyzed by referring to the video.

4) Examination of EMG Measurement Results for Intentional Tuning of Expression

Figure 7 demonstrates how the expression changes at the posing end (for subject A) and receiving end (for subject B) during the intentional tuning of expression.

The reaction velocity was measured from when the subject presents an expression and the observer reacts to the expression. From a total of 18 interactions, a mean reaction time of 423.7 ms was derived, along with a variance of 115.8. In addition, verification of the timing of the movement of eyes (orbicularis oculi) and mouth (lower orbicularis oris) revealed that the change occurred almost simultaneously, as shown in the figure.

A system exists to code the coordination of facial muscle activity that was developed by tracking the movements of each part of the face using image-processing technology (Hirayama, Kawashima, Nishiyama and Matsuyama, 2007). An "Intentional smile" and "spontaneous smile" were compared by means of this image-processing technology, and it was found that various parts of the face begin to move at the same time in the case of an "intentional smile". Our experimental results are consistent with their findings. In addition, the response time in our experimental results for a subject to mirror an observed "intentional smile" ("intentional smile" to "intentional smile") was similar to that found previously through the image-processing technology described above.

5) EMG Measurement during Tuning of Expression That Occurs Unconsciously

Figure 8 summarizes that the state of expression changes during the tuning of expression that occurs unconsciously. By referring to the video, the state of potential change for each mimetic muscle was verified. From a total of 20 tuning trials, a mean response rate of 387.2ms was derived and the variance was 294.2. This indicates that a more rapid response was found when the tuning of expression was developed unconsciously compared to when it was developed consciously. In general, major and lower orbicularis oris muscles of the talking subject showed strong activity when they were asked to talk freely. It was observed that the mimetic muscles of the observer also showed some activities.

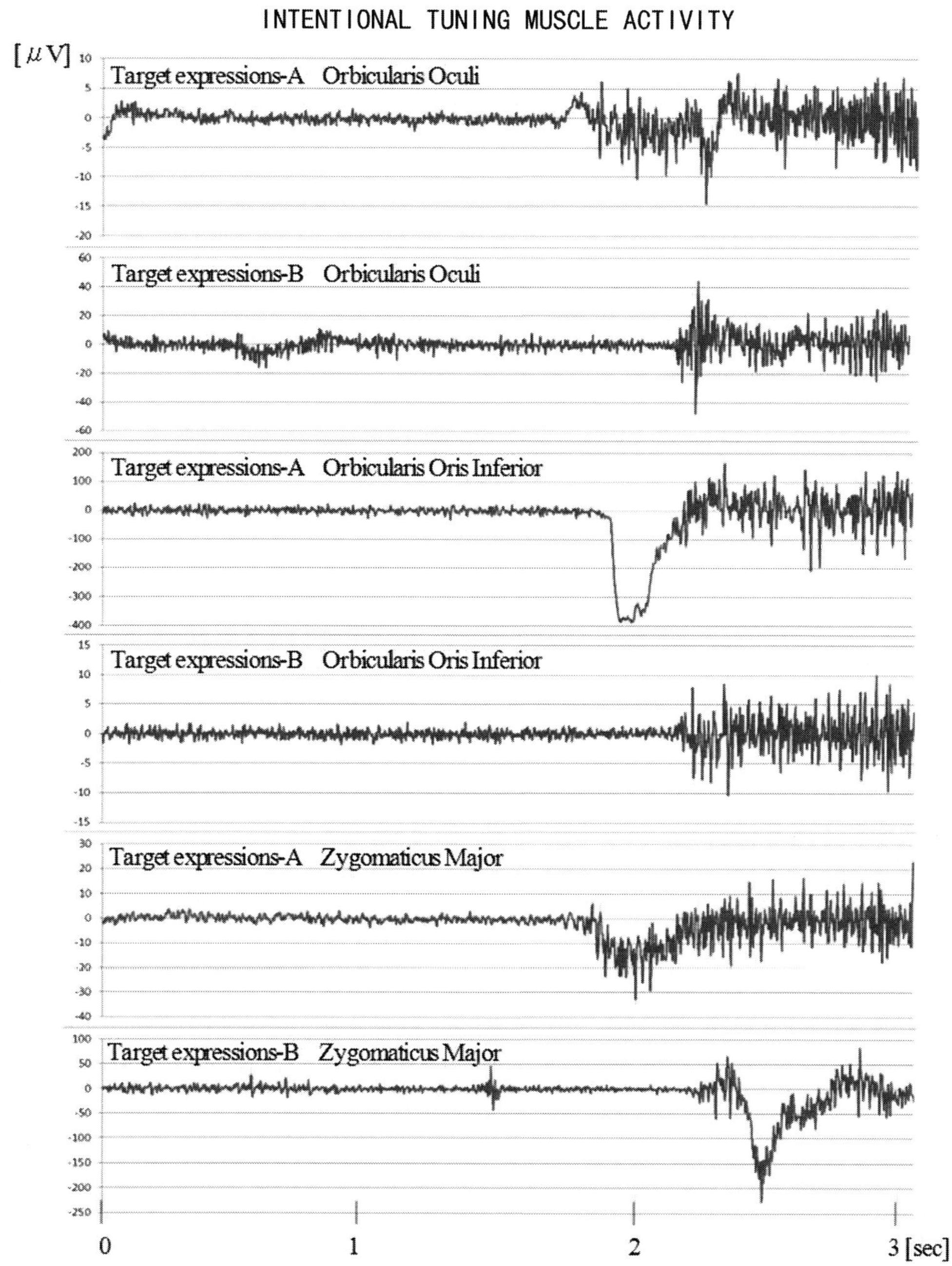

Figure 7. Changes in expression of presenter and responder during the intentional tuning of expression.

In particular, Orbicularis Oculi, Orbicularis Oris Inferior and Zygomaticus Major muscles showed strong activities when the subjects smiled and laughed out loud. In the aforementioned previous study (Hirayama, Kawashima, Nishiyama and Matsuyama, 2007) employing image processing investigations, when a subject exhibited a "spontaneous smile", the Zygomaticus Major muscle began to move faster than the other observed facial expression muscles, and the Zygomaticus Major muscle activity was larger relative to an intentional smile. In human interactions, response time in the formation of a spontaneous smile is thought to be a factor in the development of an impression of a person presenting the spontaneous smile (Matsuyama, Kawashima and Hirayama, 2009).

The individual differences observed in the response time of Zygomaticus Major muscle activity to form a spontaneous smile is a point of interest and warrants further investigation. In our investigation the activity of the Orbicularis Oris Inferior muscle was observed during conversation.

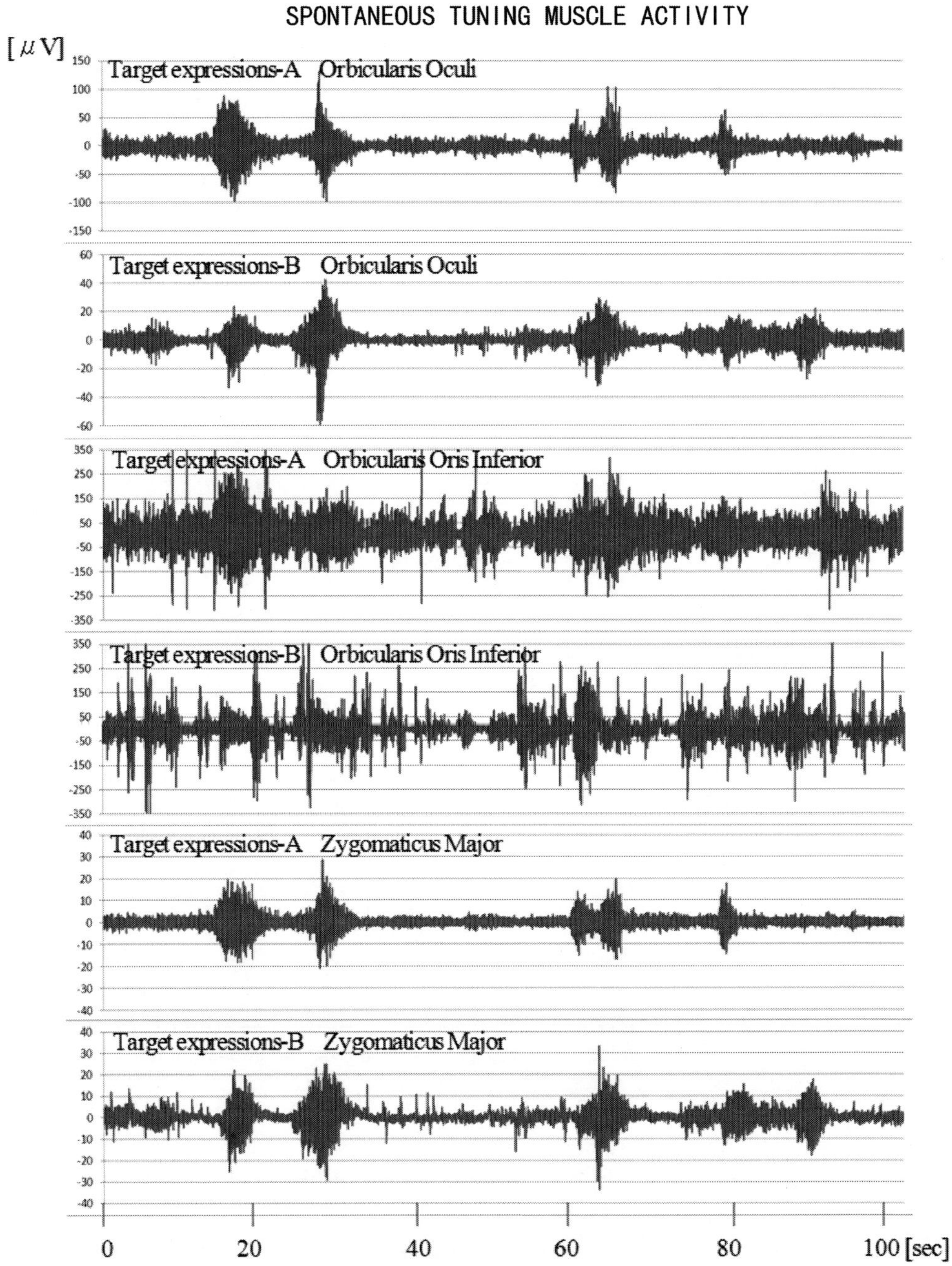

Figure 8. Change in expression during the tuning of expression that occurs spontaneously.

Muscle activation to facilitate conversation may well have impacted muscle activity during facial expression formation so it may be informative to carry out further observations in the absence of conversation.

Conclusion

Using Japanese male university students as subjects in this study, EMG of each their facial muscles (Corrugator Supercilii, Orbicularis Oculi, Levator Labii Superioris, Orbicularis Oris Inferior, Zygomaticus Major, and Masseter) were examined for the exhibition of Ekman's six expressions (happiness, surprise, sadness, anger, disgust, fear). As a result, a special characteristic in electrical potential activities was found in each mimetic muscle for each expression. EMG of facial muscles were measured during the tuning of expression while subjects communicated freely in pairs. Differences in the movement of facial muscles and in the timing were observed between intentional and unconscious tuning of expression. Future tasks include increasing the number of subjects and seeking cooperation from Japanese female university students as well as non-Japanese students (foreign students).

Acknowledgments

This work was supported by KAKENHI (Grant-in-Aid for Scientific Research (B): 21330151, Scientific Research (C): 21610007, and Research Activity Start-up: 22830033).

References

Doherty R. W. (1997). The emotional contagion scale: A measure of individual differences. *Journal of Nonverbal Behavior*, *Vol.21*, pp.131-154.

Ekman, P. and Friesen. W. V. (1975). *Unmasking the face: A guide to recognizing emotions from facial expressions*. Englewood Cliffs, NJ: Prentice Hall.

Ekman P. and Friesen W. V. (1978), *Facial Action Coding System: A technique for the measurement of facial movement,* Palo Alto, CA: Consulting Psychologists Press.

Fridlund A. J. and Cacioppo J. T. (1986). Guideline for human Electromyographic Research, *Psychophysiology*, *Vol.23* (5), pp.567-589.

Gump, B. B., Kulik, J. A. (1997). Stress, affiliation and emotional contagion. *Journal of Personality and Social Psychology*, *Vol.72* (*2*), pp.305-319.

Hatfield E., Cacioppo J. T., and Rapson R. L. (1992). Primitive emotional contagion. In M. S. Clark (Ed.), *Emotion and social behavior*: *Vol.14*. *Review of personality and social psychology* (pp.151-177). Newbury Park, CA: Sage.

Hirayama T., Kawashima H., Nishiyama M. and Matsuyama T. (2007). Facial Expression Representation based on Timing Structures in Faces. *The Transactions of Human Interface Society*, *Vol.9* (*2*), pp.271-281.

Hoffman M. L. (1987). The contribution of empathy to justice and moral judgment. In N. Eisenberg and J. Strayer (Eds.), *Empathy and its development* (pp.47-80), Cambridge, UK: Cambridge University Press.

Lundqvist, L. O. (1995) Facial EMG reactions to facial expressions: A case of facial emotional contagion? *Scandinavian Journal of Psychology*, Vol.36 (2), pp.130-141.

Matsuyama T, Kawashima H. and Hirayama T. (2009). Kansei Information Processing for the Sense of Time : Toward Enriching Human Communications, *The Journal of the Institute of Electronics, Information and Communication Engineers*, *Vol.92* (*11*), pp.952-954.

Nakamura M. (1991). Display and Decoding Rules in the Communication of Emotion: an Conceptual Analysis and a Cross-Cultural Questionnaire Study, *Bulletin 17: Graduate School of Human Sciences, Osaka University*, *Vol.17*, pp115-145.

Sonnby-Borgström M., Jönsson P., and Svensson O. (2003). Emotional empathy as related to mimicry reactions at different levels of information processing. *Journal of Nonverbal Behavior*, *Vol.27* (1), pp.3-23.

Sonnby-Borgström M., Jönsson P., and Svensson O. (2008). Gender differences in facial imitation and verbally reported emotional contagion from spontaneous to emotionally regulated processing levels. *Scandinavian Journal of Psychology*, *Vol.49* (2), pp.111-122.

Tomkins, S. S. (1962). *The positive affects: Vol.1. Affect,* imagery, and consciousness. New York: Springer Publishing.

Tomkins, S. S. (1963). *The* negative *affects: Vol.2. Affect, imagery*, and consciousness. New York: Springer Publishing.

In: Electromyography
Editor: Hiroki Takada

ISBN: 978-1- 62081-717-9

Chapter VIII

Simultaneous Measurement of Electromyogram and Near Infrared Spectroscopy during the Mastication

***Matsuura Yasuyuki*[1*], *Miyao Masaru*[2] *and Takada Hiroki*[3]**
[1]Headquarters for Innovative Society-Academia Cooperation, University of Fukui, Japan
[2]Graduate School of Information Science, Nagoya University, Japan
[3]Graduate School of Engineering, University of Fukui, Japan

Abstract

The physiological obesity-preventive mechanism of an increase in the chewing frequency has recently being clarified, and its hygienic practice has been reported. Masticatory movement is not only investigated with regard to its involvement in health promotion, but it is also attracting attention as a factor influencing the development and maintenance of brain function. Chewing training is useful for not only middle-aged and elderly obese persons, but also instruction in education at health centers and schools. In this chapter, to clarify the influence of masticatory movement on the brain, young males chewed gum, and electromyograms (EMG) of the masticatory muscles and Near - infrared spectroscopy (NIRS) were simultaneous conducted to investigate the relationship between chewing and local cerebral blood flow. It was suggested that chewing gum reduces stress.

Introduction

Histamine is released as the chewing frequency increases and acts on the satiety center in the brain (Fujise et al., 1998). Histamine also inhibits fat synthesis from glucose (Masaki et al., 2001) and promotes visceral lipolysis (Masaki et al., 2003). A physiological obesity-preventive mechanism has recently being clarified, and its hygienic practice has been reported

* E-mail: matuura@u-fukui.ac.jp.

(Ookuma et al., 2000) (Veyrune et al., 2008). In addition, masticatory movement is not only investigated with regard to its involvement in health promotion, but it is also attracting attention as a factor influencing the development and maintenance of brain function (Paulson et al., 1990) (Fisher et al., 2008). The relationship between chewing and brain function is attracting increasing attention. Reportedly, chewing is not a mere voluntary movement to move the teeth and jaws, but it is established involving advanced integrative function in the brain. With the recent development of noninvasive brain activity measurement techniques, such as functional magnetic resonance imaging (fMRI) and near-infrared spectroscopy (NIRS), and down-sizing of the devices, brain science has rapidly developed and various brain dynamics have being elucidated.

In this chapter, to clarify the influence of masticatory movement on the brain, young males chewed gum, and electromyography (EMG) of the masticatory muscles and NIRS were simultaneously performed to investigate the relationship between chewing and local cerebral blood flow.

Electromyography of the Masticatory Muscles

During mastication, the jaw contracts at a pace that results from a complex interaction between cortical descending neural pathways, a central pattern generator (CPG) located in the pons and medulla, and peripheral feedbacks arising from the teeth, the periodontal ligaments, the facial bones, the oral mucosa, the jaw muscles, and the temporomandibular joints (Lavigne et al.,1987; Lund, 1991; Nakamura and Katakura, 1995; Yamashita et al., 1999; Türker, 2002; Kolta et al., 2007). The CPG generates an intrinsic rhythm, and the chewing contractions are then modulated according to the physical properties of the food (Lund and Kolta, 2006).

Surface electromyography of the masticatory muscles is capable of noninvasively measuring muscle activity when chewing food in humans (Plesh et al., 1986; Van der Bilt et al., 1995; Van der Bilt et al., 2006). It is also attracting attention as a method of measuring the load and intensity of chewing because the frequency, duration, and intensity of chewing by the masticatory muscles can be numerically compared (Plesh et al., 1986; Lassauzay et al., 2000; Foster et al., 2006).

The masticatory muscles subjected to measurement are generally mouth-closing muscles, such as the masseter and temporal muscles used to close the jaws and clench. Electromyograms (EMG) of the mouth-opening, tongue, and cheek muscles may also be measured.

Previous findings regarding chewing activity have been obtained mainly from studies in animal models or human participants in an experimental/ laboratory setting—a major limitation, since laboratory conditions may influence masticatory parameters (Plesh et al., 1988). Furthermore, studies involving humans have mostly investigated chewing patterns during gum chewing, which is not representative of natural chewing (Van der Bilt et al., 1995). Therefore, little information currently exists on the chewing function in the natural environment.

Portable EMG recorders have been developed and used successfully to gather data on the chewing function (Gallo et al., 1999; Farella et al., 2005), and an algorithm for the automated detection of rhythmic masticatory muscle activity from EMG signals was developed and validated (Farella et al., 2009).

This algorithm allows for time-frequency analysis of rhythmic episodes and is especially suitable for investigating the features of chewing activity as it occurs in the natural environment.

The action potential of the mouth-closing muscles on surface electromyography appears in each clenching motion, but no potential appears at rest or while opening the jaws. Thus, the chewing frequency and time can be calculated by analyzing the amplitude of the EMG and duration of muscle activity on each chewing action. A disadvantage of masticatory muscle electromyography is that variation among individuals is larger than that among foods, for which standardization using a reference texture is necessary in each subject. Food texture described here represents mechanical properties, mainly hardness, cohesiveness, viscosity, elasticity, and adherence. Methods employed in reports on electromyographic analysis of masticatory movement include those adopting the cycle time or integrated value of each cycle as a representative value, dividing the period from the initiation of chewing through swallowing into early, middle, and late phases of chewing for analysis, and continuously analyzing all strokes.

Near - Infrared Spectroscopy (NIRS)

NIRS is less restrictive for examinees compared to other brain function imaging methods, such as positron emission tomography (PET) and fMRI, and fixation of the head and recumbence on a special device during measurement are unnecessary (Villringer A. and Dirnagl U., 1995) (Villringer A. and Chance B., 1997) (Okamoto et al., 2000).

However, measured values of NIRS represent relative changes in the concentration, and are not absolute values, because the optical path length from irradiation through detection cannot be measured.

When a brain region is active, blood flow increases in the region. Thus, the activity of cerebral regions can be estimated by measuring changes in cerebral blood flow. In NIRS, blood flow is determined by measuring hemoglobin carrying oxygen consumed by cell activity. In NIRS, the cerebral cortex activity is measured employing multichannel reflected light measurement on the scalp. In this method, light transmission and receiver probes are attached to the scalp. Markedly biological tissue-penetrable near infrared light at about 700-1,000 nm is irradiated from the light transmission probe, and scattered and reflected light on the cerebral cortex surface are detected through the light receiver probe.

The cerebral cortex is located at an about 15-20-mm depth from the scalp, and nerve activities and capillary blood vessels are abundant. Therefore, the cerebral cortex is appropriate for the measurement of changes in the blood hemoglobin level in the brain accompanying brain activity. The cerebral cortex is also closely connected to brain functions, such as movement, sensation, speech, and cognition.

There are 2 types of blood hemoglobin: oxygen-bound oxidized hemoglobin (Oxy-Hb) and oxygen-unbound deoxidized hemoglobin (Deoxy-Hb), and the absorbance wavelength characteristics are different. Utilizing these properties, blood flow is calculated from the attenuation level of detected light.

Measurement employing NIRS utilizes 2 characteristics of near infrared light (700-900 nm wavelengths): (a) high biological penetrability (penetration of the skin and bone), and (b) differences in the light absorption property between Oxy-Hb and Deoxy-Hb in blood.

When the scalp is irradiated with near infrared light, the light component disperses into the brain tissue due to the characteristics (a) and reaches the cerebral cortex located at an about 20-30-mm depth from the scalp (Watanabe, Murota, and Nakajima, 2005). When light is measured at a site 3 cm from the irradiated point, diffuse reflection can be detected due to the characteristics (b) (Villringer A. and Chance B., 1997).

In NIRS, Oxy-Hb, Deoxy-Hb, and the total hemoglobin level (Total-Hb) combining these in the cerebral cortex are estimated from detected light (Villringer A. and Dirnagl U., 1995) (Villringer A. and Chance B., 1997).

Since changes in each Hb measured by NIRS are relative to the baseline at measurement initiation, and the optical path length of the near infrared laser light varies depending on the physical characteristics of the subjects, it is difficult to simply compare the measured value among the subjects and calculate the mean.

Simultaneous Measurement of Masticatory Muscle EMG and NIRS

We performed the following experiment to provide an example of the influence of masticatory movement on the brain. Using NIRS and surface electromyography, chewing muscle activity and local cerebral blood flow were simultaneously measured and the influence of chewing on brain activity was evaluated. The subjects were 6 young healthy males aged 21-24 years (mean± standard deviation: 22.0±1.26 years) with no stomatognathic function abnormality, such as a defective tooth, pain of the temporomandibular joint or muscles, or disturbance of mouth opening. A temporal muscle EMG and the cerebral blood flow while chewing were simultaneously recorded. The experiment was fully explained to the subjects beforehand, and written consent was obtained. The experiment was approved by the Ethics Committee of Nagoya University Graduate School of Information Science.

The temporal muscle EMG was recorded using a multichannel telemeter system, WEB-7000 (Nihon Kohden), at a sampling frequency of 1 KHz. The measurement sites of the temporal muscle were set by assigning 1 ch each to the bilateral temples (2-ch measurement) (Figure 1).

Changes in the blood oxygenized hemoglobin level in the brain were measured using a near infrared light brain function imaging system, FOIRE-3000 (Shimadzu Corporation), at a sampling frequency of 7.7 Hz. A head holder was attached to the subject's head, and light transmission/receiver probes were attached as shown in Figure 2. Cerebral blood flow was determined in the frontal lobe employing 22-ch measurement (Figure 1).

The experiment was performed in a sitting position. After resting for 5 minutes, regarding a 20-second pre-rest, 30-second chewing, and 40-second post-rest as one set, the subject held 2 pieces of xylitol gum in their mouth in the pre-rest of the first set and repeated 3 sets, and removed the gum in the post-rest of the 3rd set. This 3-set test was repeated 3 times, and the subjects finally rested for 3 minutes (Figure 3).

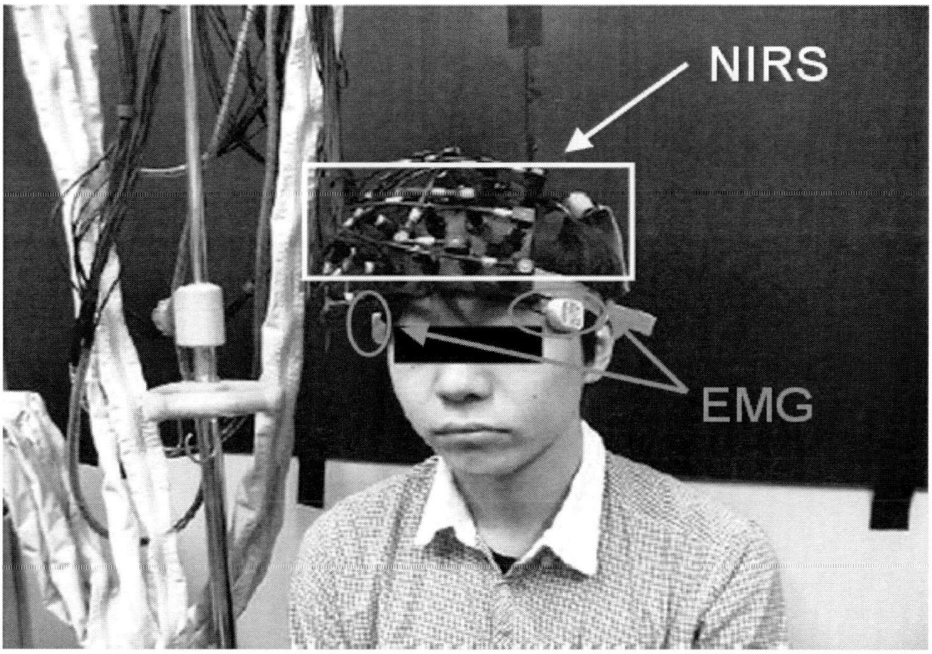

Figure 1. The setup of the experiment.

The brain activity was measured using NIRS while confirming the chewing motion in the EMG. We paid attention to the prefrontal area which controls higher thinking and judgment. The prefrontal area is involved in psychological activities, such as control of memory and emotion and inhibition of behavior. This area is also considered to be readily influenced by stress. In the analysis, 19 ch (right region of the prefrontal area), 20 ch (right central region of the prefrontal area), 21 ch (left central region of the prefrontal area), and 22 ch (left region of the prefrontal area) were used.

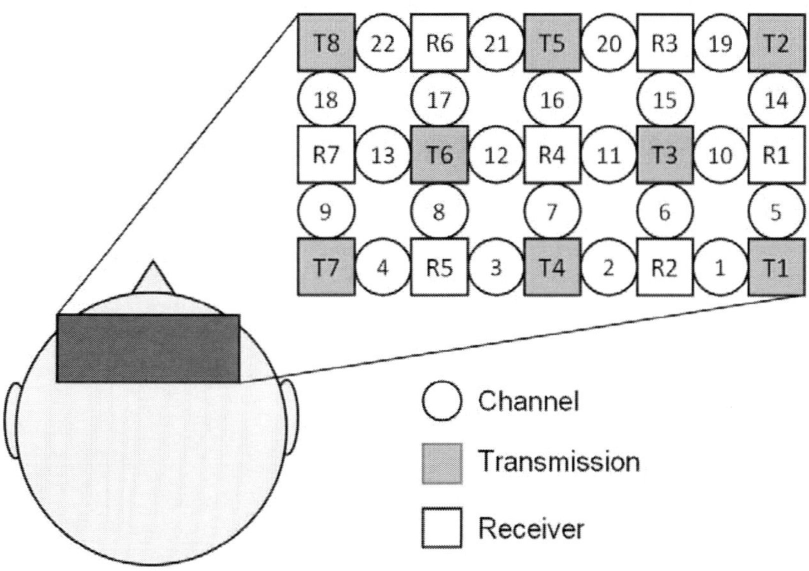

Figure 2. Arrangements of channels between transmission and receiver probes.

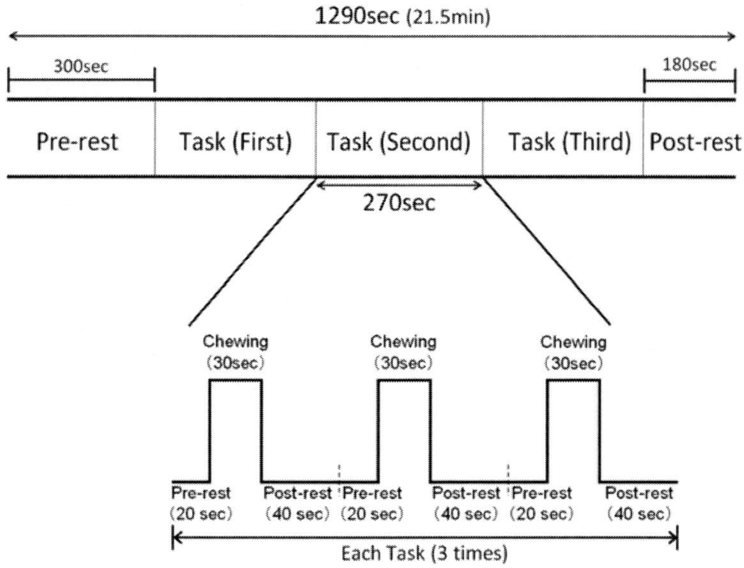

Figure 3. Experimental protocol.

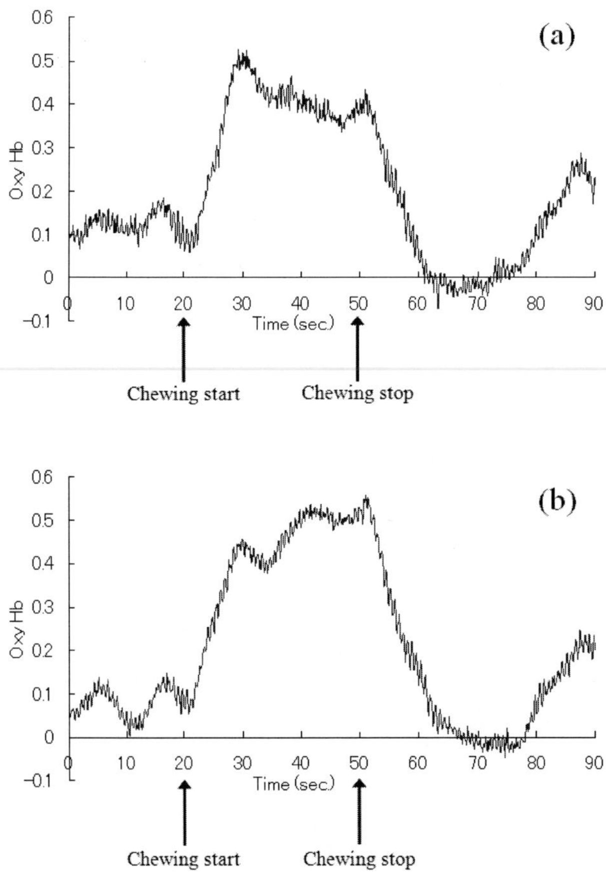

Figure 4. Averaged time courses of Oxy-Hb measured at (a) ch19, (b) ch22.

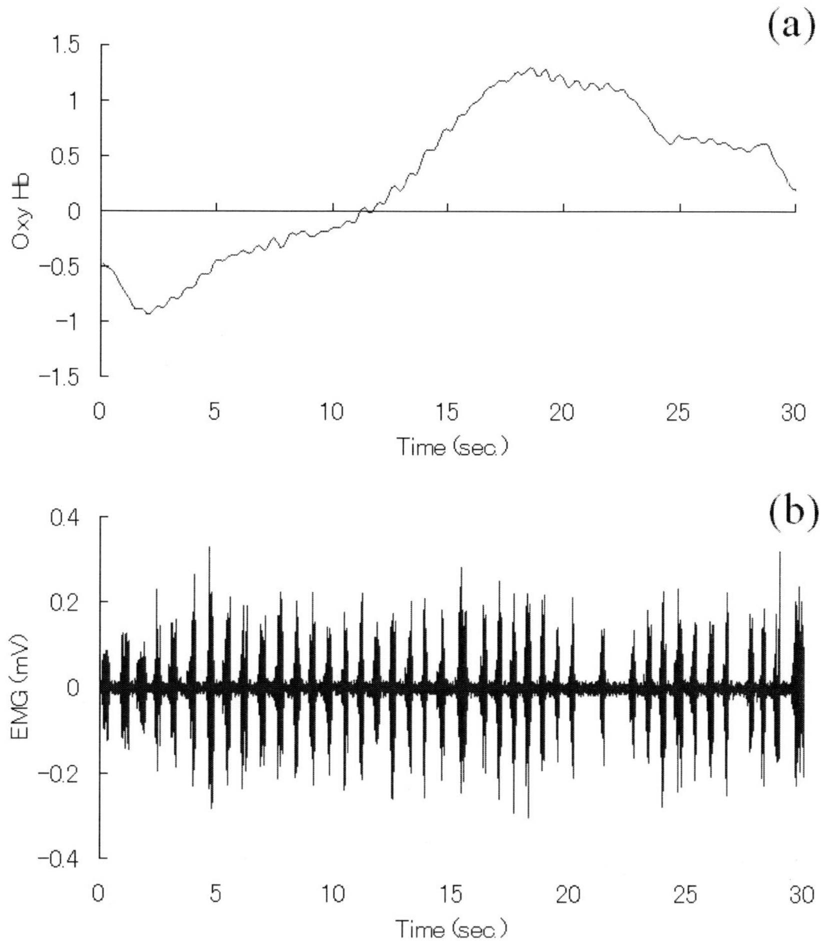

Figure 5. Time series data (a) local cerebral blood flow (Oxy-Hb), (b) EMG of the masticatory muscles.

The measured values of NIRS are relative changes in the hemoglobin level at each channel. Changes in Oxy-Hb show a particularly strong correlation with changes in the local cerebral blood flow (Hoshi Y, Kobayashi N, Tamura M, 2001) because a large amount of oxygen and nutrition are necessary for nerve activity, and changes in local blood flow reflect changes in nerve activity in the local region (Jueptner C. and Weiller C., 1995).

To control variation among the subjects, the measured values were standardized to adjust the mean and standard deviation to 0 and 1 at each channel, respectively. In addition, paying attention to changes in Oxy-Hb, we compared changes in Oxy-Hb between those at rest and during the task at each channel employing 2 way-layout ANOVA. When Oxy-Hb significantly changed during the task ($p<0.05$), it was regarded as a significant change during the task at the channel. On 2 way-layout ANOVA of the hemoglobin levels at rest and during the task, a main effect was noted in each factor ($p<0.05$). The mean Oxy-Hb in all subjects was changed by chewing (Figure 4). Chewing gum and the intensity could be confirmed in the simultaneously measured masticatory EMGs (Figure 5).

Regarding changes in Oxy-Hb, high values were detected for 5 seconds from 10 seconds after chewing initiation at the 19 and 22 ch set in the right and left regions of the prefrontal area, respectively. At the 21 ch set in the left central region of the prefrontal area, a high value was detected from 20 seconds after chewing initiation until 5 seconds after chewing completion, showing that cerebral blood flow increased while chewing but it slowly decreased after chewing and returned to the condition before chewing. Based on these findings, chewing activates the brain. It was also suggested that chewing is effective for improving memory and reducing stress.

Conclusion

To clarify the influence of masticatory movement on the brain, young males chewed gum and electromyography of the masticatory muscles and NIRS were simultaneously performed to investigate the relationship between chewing and local cerebral blood flow. Cerebral blood flow increased with chewing gum but decreased after chewing and returned to the level before chewing. The increased cerebral blood flow indicated that chewing gum activated the whole prefrontal area. It was suggested that chewing activates the brain, which may be effective for improving memory and reducing stress.

References

Farella M., Michelotti A., Carbone G., Gallo L.M., Palla S. and Martina R. (2005). Habitual daily masseter activity of subjects with different vertical craniofacial morphology. *Eur. J. Oral Sci.,* 113, 380-385.

Farella M., Palla S. and Gallo L.M. (2009). Time-frequency analysis of rhythmic masticatory muscle activity. *Muscle Nerve* 39, 828-836.

Fisher J. P., Ogoh S., Young C. N., Raven P. B. and Fadel P. J. (2008). Regulation of Middle Cerebral Artery Blood Velocity during Dynamic Exercise in Humans: Influence of Aging, *Journal of Applied Physiology,* 105, 266-273.

Fujise T., Yoshimatsu H., Kurokawa M., Oohara A., Kang M., Nakata M. and Sakata T. (1988). Satiation and Masticatory Function Modulated by Brain Histamine in Rats. *Proceedings of the Society for Experimental Biology and Medicine*, 217, 228-234.

Foster K.D., Woda A. and Peyron M.A. (2006). Effect of texture of plastic and elastic model foods on the parameters of mastication. *J. Neurophysiol.* 95, 3469-3479.

Gallo L.M., Gross S.S. and Palla S. (1999). Nocturnal masseter EMG activity of healthy subjects in a natural environment. *J. Dent. Res.,* 78, 1436-1444.

Hoshi Y., Kobayashi N. and Tamura M. (2001). Interpretation of near-infrared spectroscopy signals: a study with a newly developed perfused rat brain model. *Journal of Applied Physiology*, 90, 1657-1662.

Jueptner M. and Weiller C. (1995). Doesmeasurement of regional cerebral blood flow reflects synapticactivity? - *Implications for PET and fMRI, Neuroimage*, 2, 148-156.

Kolta A., Brocard F., Verdier D. and Lund J.P. (2007). A review of burst generation by trigeminal main sensory neurons. *Arch. Oral Biol.*, 52, 325-328.

Lassauzay C., Peyron M.A., Albuisson E., Dransfield E. and Woda A .(2000). Variability of the masticatory process during chewing of elastic model foods. *Eur. J. Oral Sci.* 108, 484-492.

Lavigne G., Kim J.S., Valiquette C. and Lund J.P. (1987). Evidence that periodontal pressoreceptors provide positive feedback to jaw closing muscles during mastication. *J. Neurophysiol.*, 58, 342-358.

Lund J.P. (1991). Mastication and its control by the brain stem. Crit Rev Oral Biol Med, 2, 33-64.

Lund J.P. and Kolta A. (2006). Generation of the central masticatory pattern and its modification by sensory feedback. *Dysphagia*, 21, 167-174.

Masaki T., Chiba S., Yoshimichi G., Yasuda T., Noguchi H., Kakuma T., Sakata T., and Yoshimatsu H. (2003). Neuronal histamine regulates food intake, adiposity, and uncoupling protein expression in agouti yellow (A(y)/a) obese mice. *Endocrinology*. 144, 2741-2748.

Masaki T., Yoshimatsu H., Chiba S., Watanabe T. and Sakata T. (2001). Central infusion of histamine reduces fat accumulation and upregulates UCP family in leptinresistant obese mice. *Diabetes*, 50, 376-384.

Nakamura Y. and Katakura N. (1995). Generation of masticatory rhythm in the brainstem. *Neurosci. Res.*, 23, 1-19.

Okamoto M., Dan H., Sakamoto K., Takeo K., Shimizu K., Kohno S., Oda I., Isobe S., Suzuki T., Kohyama K. and Dan I. (2004). Three-dimensional probabilistic anatomical cranio-cerebral correlation via the international 10-20 system oriented for transcranial functional brain mapping. *Neuroimage*, 21(1), 99-111.

Ookuma K., Yoshimatsu H., Skata T. and Adachi K. (2000). The Effect of Chewing Chart Recording in the Treatment of Obesity. *Jpn. J. Psychosom. Med.*, 40, 247-253.

Paulson O. B., Strandgaard S. and Edvinsson L. (1990). Cerebral autoregulation, *Cerebrovascular and brain metabolism reviews*, 2, 161-192.

Plesh O., Bishop B. and McCall W. (1986). Effect of gum hardness on chewing pattern. *Exp. Neurol.*, 92, 502-512.

Plesh O., Bishop B. and McCall W. (1988). Comparison of automatic and voluntary chewing patterns and performance. *Exp. Neurol.*, 99, 326-341.

Tamura T., Eda H., Takada M. and Kubodera T. (1989). New instrument for monitoring hemoglobin oxygenation. *Advances in Experimental Medicine and Biology*, 248, 103-107.

Türker K.S. (2002). Reflex control of human jaw muscles. *Crit. Rev. Oral Biol. Med.*, 13, 85-104.

Van der Bilt A., Engelen L., Pereira L. J., Van der Glas H.W. and Abbink J.H. (2006). Oral physiology and mastication. *Physiol. Behav.*, 89, 22-27.

Van der Bilt A., Weijnen F.G., Ottenhoff F.A.M., Van der Glas H.W. and Bosman F. (1995). The role of sensory information in the control of rhythmic open-close movements in humans. *J. Dent. Res.*, 74, 1658-1664.

Veyrune J.L., Chaussain Miller C., Czernichow S., Ciangura C.A., Nicolas E. and Hennequin M. (2008). Impact of Morbid Obesity on Chewing Ability. *Obesity Surgery*, 18(11), 1467-1472.

Villringer A. and Chance B. (1997). Non-invasive optical spectroscopy and imaging of human brain function. *Trends Neurosci.,* 20, 435–442.

Villringer A. and Dirnagl U. (1995). Coupling of brain activity and cerebral blood flow: basis of functional neuroimaging. *Cerebrovasc. Brain Metab. Rev.*, 7, 240–276.

Yamashita S., Hatch J.P. and Rugh J.D. (1999). Does chewing performance depend upon a specific masticatory pattern? *J. Oral Rehabil.,* 26, 547-553.

In: Electromyography
Editor: Hiroki Takada

ISBN: 978-1- 62081-717-9

Chapter IX

Visualizing EMG and Heart Rate Synchronized with Human Motion Based on 3DCG

***Tsuyoshi Matsukawa*[1*] *and Kiyoko Yokoyama*[2]**
[1]Faculty of Information Science,
Aichi Institute of Technology, Yakusa-cho, Japan
[2]Graduate School of Design and Architecture,
Nagoya City University, Chikusa, Japan

Abstract

In this chapter, a new method for visualizing bio-information. In this visualization, 3DCG avatar motion represents human motion captured with high accuracy by an optical motion capture system. EMG and heart rate are represented by the color or size of avatar organs. The characteristic of the proposed method is intuitive recognition of health conditions. In this visualization, multiple biosignals can be used and health conditions of a number of people can be represented. The visualization method can apply to synchronized analysis of muscle activity, heart rate variability and motion.

Introduction

Three-dimensional imaging techniques in medical science are applied to visualize non-observable organs or tissues for diagnosis and treatment. Examples of such techniques are computed tomography (CT), X-ray imaging, magnetic resonance imaging (MRI), fiber scope and ultra-sonic imaging (Lysdahl and Borretzen, 2007). The balance of autonomic nervous activity, relaxation effect, sleep stage, muscle activity, and health conditions are estimated based on analysis of bio-signals. Several representation methods such as tachograms,

[*] E-mail address: matsukawa@aitech.ac.jp.

mapping charts, and tables are used for visualizing results derived from bio-signal analysis. Motion analysis is applied to sports activity, evaluation of work posture, and diagnosis of the effect of rehabilitation. Video image analysis is generally applied to motion analysis.

There are few examples of integrated analysis of biosignals and human motion. One is to analyze human motion using electromyogram (EMG) and video image. In our visualization, 3DCG avatar motion represents human motion captured with high accuracy by an optical motion capture system. Muscle activity and heart rate are represented as color or size of avatar organs. There are a few examples which represent human motion synchronized with EMG signals. In these visualizations, the representation of health conditions is inadequate, i.e. simple cylinder body model (Urawki et al., 2004; Seri et al., 2000; Inaba et al., 2006). The key characteristics of the proposed system are its highly accurate estimation of health conditions and intuitive recognition of health conditions. In this visualization, multiple biosignals can be used and the health conditions of a number of persons can be represented. The visualization method can be used for synchronized analysis of heart rate variability, muscle activity and motion. The autonomic nervous response and the muscle activity in relation to the change in transitional motion can be presented at the same time. A wide application is possible because the visualization method can present intuitive representations of health conditions in daily life for multifaceted evaluation of physiological conditions.

SEMG and ECG Visualization Synchronized with Motion

An outline showing the proposed visualizing system is presented in Figure 1. Reflection markers are captured using an optical motion capture system (EVaRT4.7: MotionAnalysis, USA) at 60 [fps: frame per second]. Human motion is estimated from the time series of marker positions. Surface electromyogram (SEMG) and electrocardiogram (ECG) are collected using a telemetric portable bio-amplifier (BA1104, TU: Digitex lab. Co., ltd, Japan) to estimate muscle activities and heart rate variability. These data are stored on a Pentium PC via a 16 [bit] A/D converter using the analogue input function of EVaRT. A sampling trigger is generated at capturing intervals by the motion capture system with a sampling frequency of 1200 [Hz].

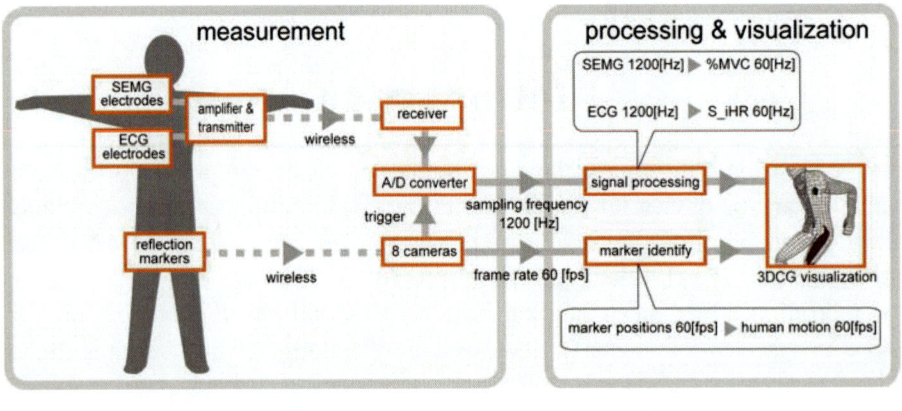

Figure 1. Outline of proposed visualizing system.

Percentage of maximum voluntary contraction (%MVC) and standardized instantaneous heart rate are used as the health condition parameters, which make easy comparison possible among a number of people without the effects of personal differences. The procedures for visualizing %MVC and standardized iHR are as follows.

1) SEMG

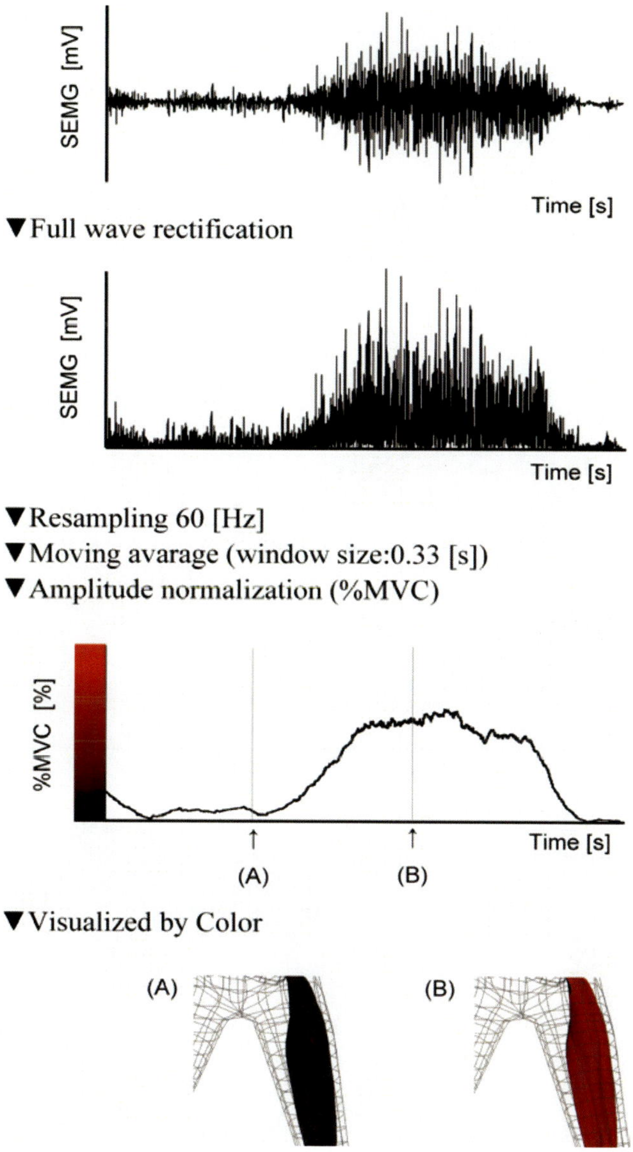

Figure 2. Method of signal processing and visualizing SEMG.

The methods used for signal processing and visualizing of SEMG are shown in Figure 2.

1) Full wave rectification is applied to the sampled SEMG signal are calculated.
2) Rectified SEMG is resampled at 60 [Hz].

3) Low-pass filter is applied to the resampled SEMG using the moving average method whose window width is 20 frames (0.33 [s]). The amplitude is defined as voluntary contraction.
4) %MVC [%], which is the rate of voluntary contraction and maximum voluntary contraction, is calculated.
5) %MVC is assigned to the tone of color of the targeted muscle. The color of the muscle model is dark when the %MVC is low (model A). On the other hand, the color of the muscle model is vivid when the %MVC is high (model B).

2) ECG

The method of signal processing and visualizing of ECG are shown in Figure 3.

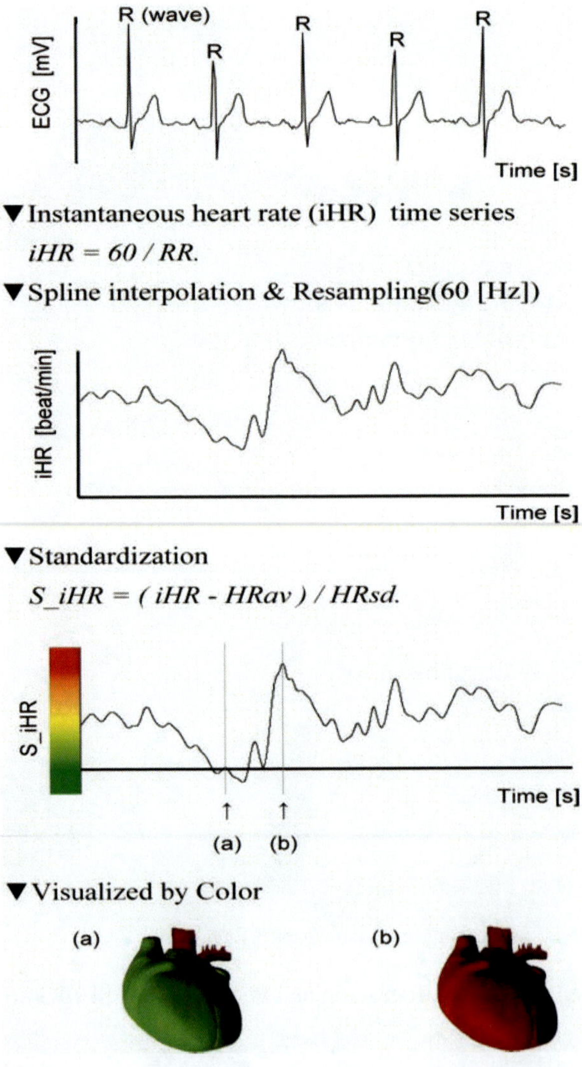

Figure 3. Method of signal processing and visualizing ECG.

1) Instantaneous heart rate (iHR [bpm: beats per minute]) is calculated from the R-R interval (RR [s]) of ECG in accordance with the following equation :

iHR = 60 / RR.

2) The iHR time series is interpolated by the spline method. This interpolated time series is resampled at 60 [Hz].
3) To calculate S_iHR, average and standard deviation are calculated from the iHR time series measured in the resting condition. S_iHR is calculated by

S_iHR = (iHR – HRave) / HRsd,

where HRave is the average and HRsd is the standard deviation of the time series of iHR during the resting condition.

4) S_iHR is assigned to the color of the heart model.Sympatho-vagal balance controls heart rate variability. Parasympathetic nerves decelerate the heart rate and sympathetic nerves accelerate it (Hainsworth, 1995). Warm color is associated with sympathetic nerves and cool color with the parasympathetic nerves. The S_iHR is neutral (average iHR of during resting condition) so the color of the left heart model (model a) is green. The S_iHR is high so the color of the right heart model (model b) is red (warm color).

Examples of Visualization

1) Aerobic Dance

Example of visualizing %MVCs and instantaneous heart rate during aerobic dance (knee-up 300 [sec]: tempo 140 [bpm]) is shown in Figure 4. Motions and health conditions at 9 [sec] after starting (left figure) and at 199 [sec] after starting (right figure) are shown. Subject is a female, who is 160cm tall and is 50kg in weight.

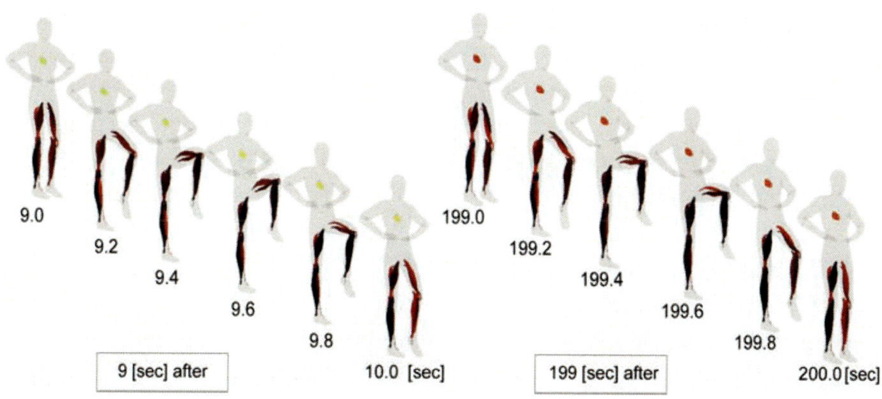

Figure 4. Visualizing example of aerobic dance.

The SEMG electrodes were positioned on the front of the thigh (vastus medialis), back of the thigh (biceps femoris), front of the shin (tibialis anterior) and back of the shin (gastrocnemius) (Zipp, 1982). These six avatars represent six motions, muscle activities and instantaneous heart rate at 0.2 [sec] intervals for 1 [sec] in this figure. Muscle color is indicated in red and black when %MVC is 0% and 40%, respectively. Color of the heart is green and red when S_iHR is 0 and 40, respectively. The muscle activities of the front thigh of the left leg and the back thigh of the right leg were respectively increased. The difference caused by continuance time was shown in knee position and in activities of the back thigh muscle of the left leg and front shin muscle of the right leg. The heart rate was increased at 199 [sec] later. But heart rates were constant from 9 [sec] to 10 [sec].

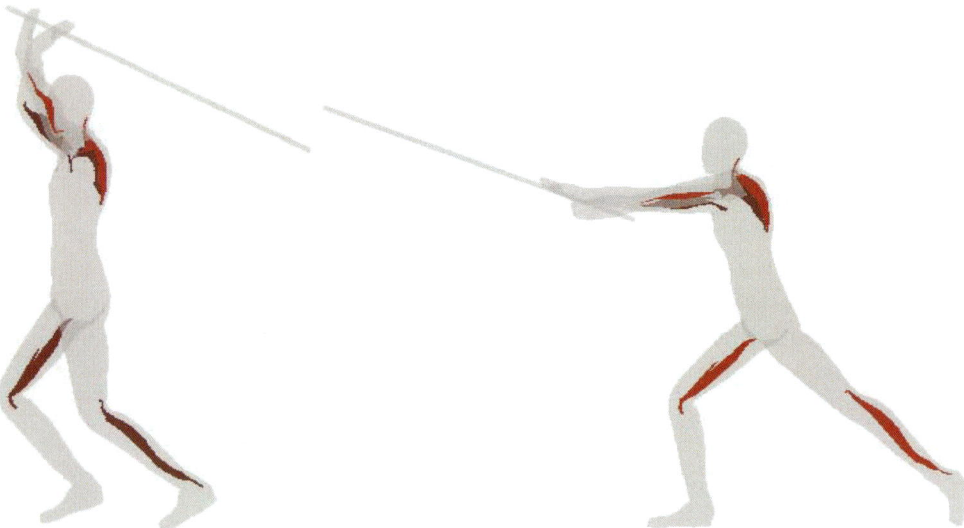

Figure 5. Visualizing example of "Kendo" motion.

The effects of aerobic dance can be intuitively presented. The muscle activities of whole leg, exercise volume reflecting heart rate and motion can be represented comprehensively.

2) "Kendo" Motion

Visualizing examples of the motion of the "Kendo" are shown in Figure 5. The motion is named "Menuchi".

The SEMG electrodes were positioned on the left and right trapezius, left brachioradialis, right biceps brachii, left tibialis anteriorfront and right hamstring muscles. The comparison with an expert and a beginner or applying to the self-learning of "Kendo" can be performed based on this kind of visualization.

3) Posture Change to Standing from Sitting

Visualizing examples of %MVC and instantaneous heart rate while changing to standing from sitting are shown in Figure 6. The instantaneous heart rate is represented by color of avatar's heart. The SEMG electrodes were positioned on the subject's left leg muscle (rectus femoris and gastrocnemius). Standing induces an increase of heart rate that follows a peculiar time course initially.

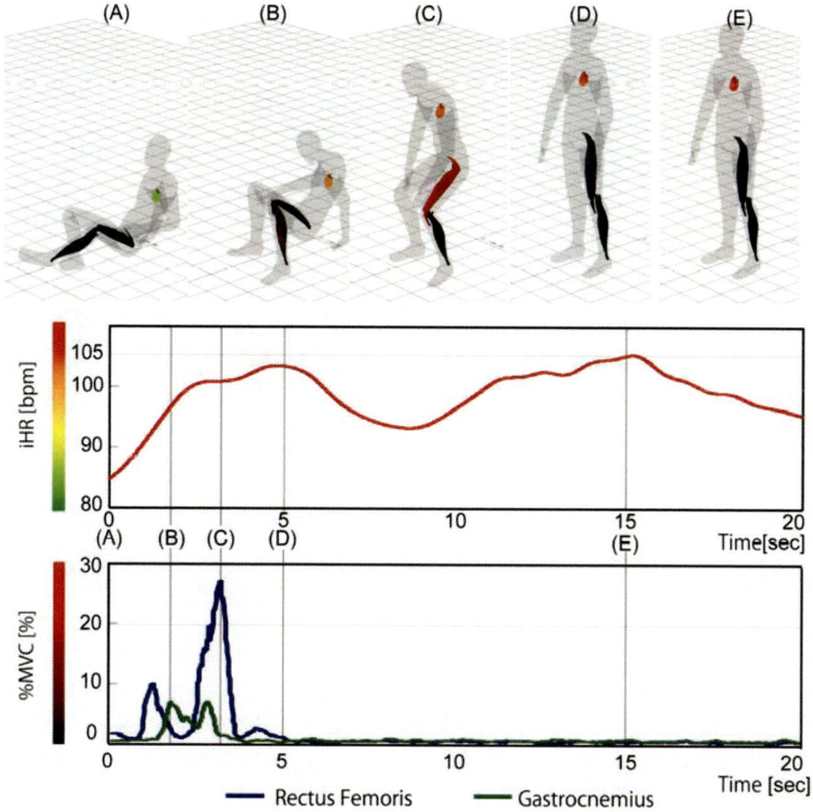

Figure 6. Snapshots of the avatar animation while transient motion from sitting to standing.

This visualization shows the change of heart rate, condition of muscle activity simultaneously immediately after standing. The relationship between the heart rate change and the muscle activities can be presented intuitively using this visualization.

4) Nurse-Care Motions

Nurse-care motions performed by two pairs are shown in Figure 7. The SEMG electrodes were positioned on the right arm muscle (biceps brachii), waist muscle (erector spinae), and right leg muscle (vastus medialis). Muscle color is indicated in red and black when %MVC is 0% and 30%, respectively.

Color of heart is green and red when S_iHR is 0 and 10, respectively. It is clear from the avatar motion seen in the figure on the right that the service person is making effective use of his/her knee motion.

The muscle activity and heart rate of the service person and the assisted person in the figure on the left were higher than in the one on the right. The mutual relationship between the assisted person and service person can be present comprehensively. The relationship between nurse-care motion and physical workload of two persons can be evaluated intuitively.

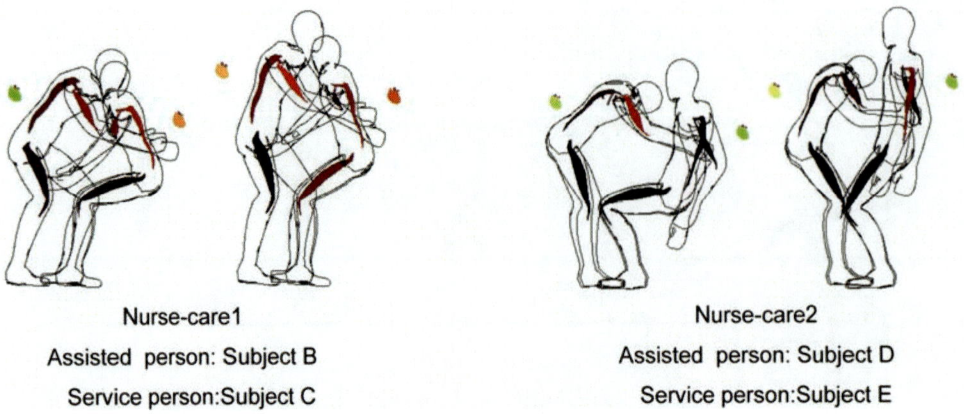

Figure 7. Visualizing example of nurse-care motions performed by two pairs.

5) Evaluation of Human Interface Usability of Control Panel

Twelve snapshots of the avatar animation representing panel operation are shown in Figure 8.

The figure shows motions operating panel and muscle activities. The height of panel is 10 [cm], 30 [cm] and 50 [cm] from the bottom in the figure. The panel degree of leaning is 0 [deg.], 30 [deg.], 60 [deg.] and 90 [deg.] from the left in the figure. In case 50 [cm]-height from sitting seat, the activity of trapezius muscle and biceps brachii muscle were high.

In case 10 [cm]-height from sitting seat, the activity of brachioradialis was high. The workload while panel operation is able to estimate intuitively.

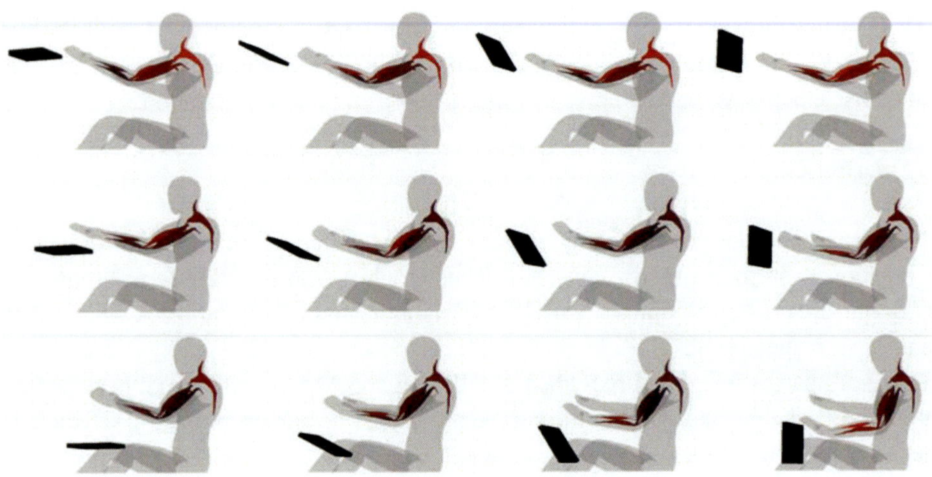

Figure 8. Snapshots of the avatar animation of operating consol panel.

Conclusion

In this chapter, a new method for visualizing SEMG, heart rate and human motion, which represents muscle activity and heart rate variability of a number of people synchronized with motion. In the experimental examples, our method can present multi physiological conditions, such as muscle activity and heart rate variability of a number of people dynamically and intuitively. This is very large merit for analysis of workload of cooperative motion compared with the conventional motion analysis method or bio-signal analysis. This system can be used as a support technology to obtain new findings in the field of ergonomics, for example in evaluating biological load in daily living activities or at production sites.

References

Hainsworth, R. The control and physiological importance of heart rate. In: Malik, M. and Camm, A. J., editors. *Heart Rate Variability*, New York: Futura Pub; 1995; 3-19.

Inaba, H., Taki, T., Miyazaki, S., Hasegawa, J., Koeda, M. and Kitagawa, K. (2006). Visual sensing in sports motion capturing. *IEICE technical report. Image engineering,* 105(500), 7-12.

Lysdahl, K. B. and Borretzen, I. (2007). Geographical variation in radiological services: a nationwide survey. *BMC Health Serv. Res.*, 7-21.

Seri, A., Yamane, K. and Nakamura, Y. (2000). Behavior capture system. *ROBOMEC'00,* 2000(3), 2A1.79.118(1)-2A1.79.118(2) (in Japanese).

Urawaki, K., Masuda, Y., Yasumuro, Y., Manabe, Y. and Chihara, K. (2004). Development of the learning environment for sports-form education with the visualization of biophysical information. *Proceedings of the 14th International Conference on Artificial Reality and Telexistence*, 576-579.

Zipp, P. (1982). Recommendation for the standardization of lead positions in surface electromyography. *European Journal of Applied Physiology*, 50(1), 41-54.

In: Electromyography
Editor: Hiroki Takada

ISBN: 978-1- 62081-717-9

Chapter X

Effects of Walking Speeds and Normalization Methods on the Muscular Activity of the Paretic Lower Limb in Stroke Subjects

Luci F. Teixeira-Salmela[1], Christina D. C. M. Faria, Marie-Hélène Milot and Sylvie Nadeau

[1] Department of Physical Therapy,
Universidade Federal de Minas Gerais, Brazil

[2] École de réadaptation, Université de Montréal and Centre de recherche interdisciplinaire en réadaptation (CRIR),
Institut de Réadaptation Gingras-Lindsay-de-Montréal, Canada

Abstract

The purpose of this chapter was to compare the magnitude of the electromyographic (EMG) signals of the paretic lower limb muscles of stroke subjects between comfortable and maximal walking speeds, considering two methods of normalization. A convenience sample of 10 chronic stroke subjects walked at their self-selected comfortable and maximal walking speeds. The EMG signals were collected from the rectus femoris, biceps femoris, tibialis anterior, and lateral gastrocnemius muscles of the paretic lower limb and were quantified by the root mean squares and normalized by the mean and peak dynamic methods. For all muscles, the ANOVA performed on the mean EMG values over specific periods of muscular activity revealed significant interactions between walking speeds and methods of normalization ($9.02<F<31.24; 0.001<p<0.016$). The effects of the methods were greatest at the maximal speeds. The inter-subject variability was also modified by the normalization method, but not consistently for all of the

[1] Address Correspondence and Request for Reprints, Professor Luci Fuscaldi Teixeira-Salmela, Department of Physical Therapy, Universidade Federal de Minas Gerais, Avenida Antônio Carlos, 6627 - Campus Pampulha, 31270-901 Belo Horizonte, Minas Gerais, Brazil, Phone : 55-31-3409-7403; Fax : 55-31-3409-4783 , E-mail: lfts@ufmg.br.

muscles, except for the rectus femoris. In general, the greatest inter-subject variability was observed at maximal walking speeds. The normalization methods and the walking speeds modified the EMG levels and the inter-subject variability. These findings should be considered when the impact of locomotor interventions on EMG values with stroke subjects is studied.

Keywords: Electromyography, stroke, gait analysis, walking speed

Introduction

Stroke is one of the most common causes of long-term disability worldwide, and is an important public health concern (Geyh *et al.*, 2004). Among all disabilities demonstrated by stroke subjects, impaired walking is considered to be one of the most important (Geyh *et al.*, 2004; Olney and Richards, 1996). It is well recognized that changes in gait performance are the greatest contributors to functional disabilities post-stroke (Jorgensen *et al.*, 1995). In addition, the degree to which walking is impaired following a stroke relates to the severity of the subjects' lower motor extremity deficiencies (Perry *et al.*, 1995) and to the degree to which community subjects are functionally independent (Wade *et al.*, 1987). Furthermore, walking is the activity which stroke subjects rate as being the most important (Bohannon *et al.*, 1988). Considering these factors, several studies have provided better comprehension of gait disturbances of stroke subjects (Olney and Richards, 1996; Jorgensen *et al.*, 1995; Perry *et al.*, 1995; Wade *et al.*, 1987; Bohannon *et al.*, 1988; Bohannon, 1992; Nadeau *et al.*, 1999; Olney *et al.*, 1994; Salbach *et al.*, 2001; Teixeira-Salmela *et al.*, 2001).

One of the most employed variables to investigate gait performance is walking speed (Olney and Richards, 1996; Bohannon, 1992; Nadeau *et al.*, 1999; Olney *et al.*, 1994; Salbach *et al.*, 2001), given its objectivity (Bohannon, 1992; Salbach *et al.*, 2001) and importance for safe ambulation (Cohen *et al.*, 1987). Another variable often used in investigations regarding gait performance is the electromyographic (EMG) activity of the lower limb muscles (Burden *et al.*, 2003; Hesse *et al.*, 2001; Olney and Richards, 1996; Yang and Winter, 1984), since the most significant impairment for gait performance is the inability to generate voluntary muscle contractions of normal magnitudes and in a coordinated manner (Olney and Richards, 1996). However, there were no studies found which compared EMG activity of the lower limb muscles between comfortable and maximal walking speeds with stroke subjects.

Another important question which has not yet been well addressed is related to the optimal normalization method of the EMG signals to be applied in gait analyses of the paretic lower limb of stroke subjects. Burden *et al.* (2003) compared four different methods of normalization of the EMG signals recorded during gait of healthy subjects, walking on a treadmill at normal speeds. Despite their important results, some questions regarding the normalization still remain. One is related to the best normalization method to analyse the muscular activity of stroke subjects during gait. This is mainly for the muscles of the paretic lower limb, which showed decreased capacity to activate motor units, as well as reduced number of functioning motor units and motor unit firing rates (Carr and Shepherd, 1998; McComas *et al.*, 1973). Unanimous agreement on EMG of the lower limb of stroke subjects is the high levels of inter-individual variability (Den Otter *et al.*, 2007; Olney and Richards,

1996). One way of addressing this problem is the investigation of the normalization methods most suitable for the reduction of variability associated with other factors in gait patterns.

Amongst the four methods of normalization which have been most investigated, two have been shown to reduce inter-individual variability: The mean and the peak dynamic methods (Burden *et al.*, 2003; Yang and Winter, 1984). Both methods have some advantages, since the normalized values are derived from walking trials (Yang and Winter, 1984).

The first aim of this chapter was to compare the magnitudes of the EMG signals of the paretic lower limb muscles of stroke subjects between comfortable and maximal walking speeds, considering two means of normalization, the mean and peak dynamic methods. The second was to describe the intra- and inter-subject variability of each method at both walking speeds. All comparisons were carried-out considering four different muscles of the paretic lower limb: The rectus femoris, lateral hamstrings (biceps femoris), tibialis anterior, and lateral gastrocnemius. At a given speed, for each muscle, the period of the gait cycle which showed the most important EMG levels, determined from the averaged EMG profiles, were considered for analyses.

Methods

Subjects

Subjects with hemiparesis due to stroke were recruited from a rehabilitation center in the Montréal area (Institut de réadaptation Gingras-Lindsay-de-Montréal). Participants required the following criteria to participate: 1) had a chronic (six months or more) unilateral stroke, 2) were able to walk 10 meters independently with or without a cane, and 3) had residual weaknesses of the paretic lower limb. The following exclusion criteria were applied: 1) use of orthoses, 2) comprehensive aphasia, 3) incontinence, 4) unstable medical conditions, 5) histories of injuries, and 6) anesthesia of the lower limbs. This information was gathered on a clinical chart, from the participants themselves, or by their proxy. Authorization by the primary care physician was obtained, if necessary. All potential participants completed an informed and written consent prior to the assessment sessions in accordance with the ethical standards of the University ethical committee.

Evaluation

Clinical Evaluations

For characterization purposes, demographic and clinical data were collected on all subjects by a trained physical therapist. Clinical data were related to the physical impairments of the lower limb evaluated by the lower extremity component (leg and foot) of the Chedoke-McMaster Stroke Assessment (Gowland *et al.*, 1993), balance (Berg Balance Scale) (Berg *et al.*, 1995), and by clinical measures of comfortable and maximal walking speeds, quantified by the five meter walking test (Salbach *et al.*, 2001).

Gait Evaluations

Gait parameters were collected during the five gait cycles at both self-selected comfortable and maximal speeds. Unilateral surface EMG signals of the following four selected muscles of the paretic lower limb were recorded during gait: The rectus femoris, biceps femoris, tibialis anterior, and lateral gastrocnemius. These muscles are recognized as the most important during gait (Olney and Richards, 1996; Winter, 1991) in studies with stroke subjects (Den Otter *et al.*, 2007; Engardt *et al.*, 1995).

Small, disposable, disc silver–silver chloride (Ag/AgCl) surface electrodes with a 13.2 mm^2 active surface area (AMBU_ Blue Sensor M), were arranged in a bipolar configuration with a two cm inter-electrode distance, and directly applied over the muscle bellies, parallel to their fiber orientation. A reference electrode was placed over the head of the fibula. Each electrode placement site was prepared using recommended preparation techniques (Cram *et al.*, 1998). The EMG cables were connected to a Noraxon Telemyo 900 portable integrated EMG multi-channel transmitter (Noraxon, Scottsdale, AZ) (weight=0.453 kg per transmitter), which was attached around the subjects' waist. All myoelectric signals underwent an analog-digital conversion before being relayed to the receiver/amplifier units. At this point, the myoelectrical signals were amplified with an overall gain of 2,000 and band-pass filtered (10–500 Hz). Finally, the signals were digitized at a sampling frequency of 1,200 Hz and stored on a computer using a custom-made Labview program (National Instruments, Austin, TX).

Electromyographic Data Processing

First, the EMG signals of all the collected gait trials were full wave rectified and band-pass filtered. All raw EMG signals were visually inspected following signal offset removal. Then, the stride characteristics of each gait cycle were determined considering the peak signals provided by the footswitches located on the soles of the shoes at the heel, metatarsal heads, and mid-foot. The EMG data were then, time normalized to 100% of the gait cycle using a two-point method. The EMG and the footswitch signals were processed by a locally developed software. Out of five collected gait trials, the three which showed the most similar values for speed, cadence, and EMG activity were averaged and selected for analyses. The normalization process of the EMG signals was performed using the mean and the peak dynamic methods. For the mean dynamic method, the mean RMS values for the complete stride of the averaged trials were calculated for each participant. For the peak dynamic method, the maximal RMS values were calculated. To allow comparisons between the magnitudes of muscular activity at the comfortable and maximal walking speeds, the EMG signals at both speeds were normalized using the mean and peak values of the comfortable walking speed. Finally, for each method and speed, the periods of the gait cycle where the EMG activity was the most important were visually identified for each muscle by careful observations and analyses of the EMG profiles (Figures 1 and 2), considering the specific phases of the gait cycle, as performed in previous studies (Den Otter *et al.*, 2004; Murray *et al.*, 1984; Shiavi *et al.*, 1987; Winter, 1991). Over each of the selected periods, the means of the EMG values obtained by each normalization method was calculated. Then, the ratio of the differences between the mean values of the two methods over the peak dynamic method, were calculated to better understand the amplitude differences between these normalization methods. The same approach was used to assess the differences between gait speeds for a given normalization method.

Statistical Analyses

Descriptive statistics (means and standard deviations) were computed for all demographic, clinical, and EMG variables and tests for normality were carried out for all investigated parameters. Two-way repeated measure ANOVAs were employed to investigate the mean and interaction effects between the walking speeds (comfortable and maximal) and the normalization methods (mean and peak). The coefficients of variation (CV), obtained by the ratio of the standard deviations to the mean values, expressed in percentages (Portney and Watkins, 2000), were used to determine the intra-subject variability for each walking speed, as well as the inter-individual variability for each method of normalization at each walking speed. All statistical analyses were performed with the SPSS® software (version 15.0) with the significance level of $\alpha<0.05$.

Results

Subjects' Characteristics

Ten hemiparetic subjects, six men and four women, with a mean age of 60±12.4 years (ranging from 46 to 78 years) and a mean time post-stroke of 62.5 ± 52.8 months (ranging from 25 to 172 months), participated. Five subjects were right side paretic. The median Chedoke scores were five and four for the leg and foot, respectively, and the Berg Balance Scale score was 53/56. During the five meter walking test, the mean comfortable walking speed was 0.82 ± 0.29 m/s (ranging from 0.41 to 1.44) and the mean maximal walking speed was 1.22 ± 0.47 m/s (ranging from 0.42 to 2.03). All subjects were able to increase their maximal walking speeds, when compared to the comfortable ones ($p\leq0.001$). During EMG data collection, the mean comfortable speed was 0.69 ± 0.30 m/s (ranging from 0.36 to 1.39) and the mean maximal walking was 1.19 ± 0.44 m/s (ranging from 0.49 to 1.71). Once again, all subjects were able to increase their maximal walking speeds, when compared to their comfortable ones ($p\leq0.001$).

Pattern Characteristics of the EMG Activity

As can be observed in Figures 1 and 2, for all muscles, the average pattern characteristics of the EMG activity were similar between the two methods of normalization, although the EMG levels and the inter-subject variability (one standard deviation) were greatest for the data normalized by the mean dynamic method. The following descriptions regarding the EMG profiles of each muscle could thus, be applied to both methods of normalization.

The patterns of the rectus femoris muscle were biphasic at both walking speeds. Considering the mean profiles, the first period of EMG activity during the gait cycle began at mid-swing (~80%) and finished before mid-stance, 20 and 30% for the maximal and comfortable speeds, respectively. The second period of activity was clearer at maximal speeds and varied from the second half of the stance to the initial swing (maximal speed: 35%-60%; comfortable speed: 50-70%). The three periods of EMG activity were selected for analyses: 0-20%, 35-70%, and 80-100% of the gait cycle. During these periods, the maximal values of the normalized EMG activities were observed just prior to the initial contact. The patterns of the biceps femoris were monophasic at both walking speeds. The period of the gait cycle of major EMG activity began at mid-swing (~75%), continued until the end of the gait cycle, and ended at the terminal stance (~35%). The highest EMG amplitudes were depicted just prior to the initial contact. For this specific muscle, two periods of EMG activity were selected for analyses: 0-35% and 75-100%. The tibialis anterior showed biphasic patterns at both walking speeds. The first period of EMG activity began at mid-swing (~80%) and continued until mid-stance (~15%). The second period was observed at the terminal stance and continued until the initial swing (comfortable speed: 45-70%; maximal speed: 40-60%). Three periods were then, selected for analyses: 0-15%, 40-70%, and 80-100%. The maximal levels of EMG activity were often observed at the initial contact. It should also be noted that this muscle had the most similar EMG patterns and amplitudes between the walking speeds (Figures 1 and 2).

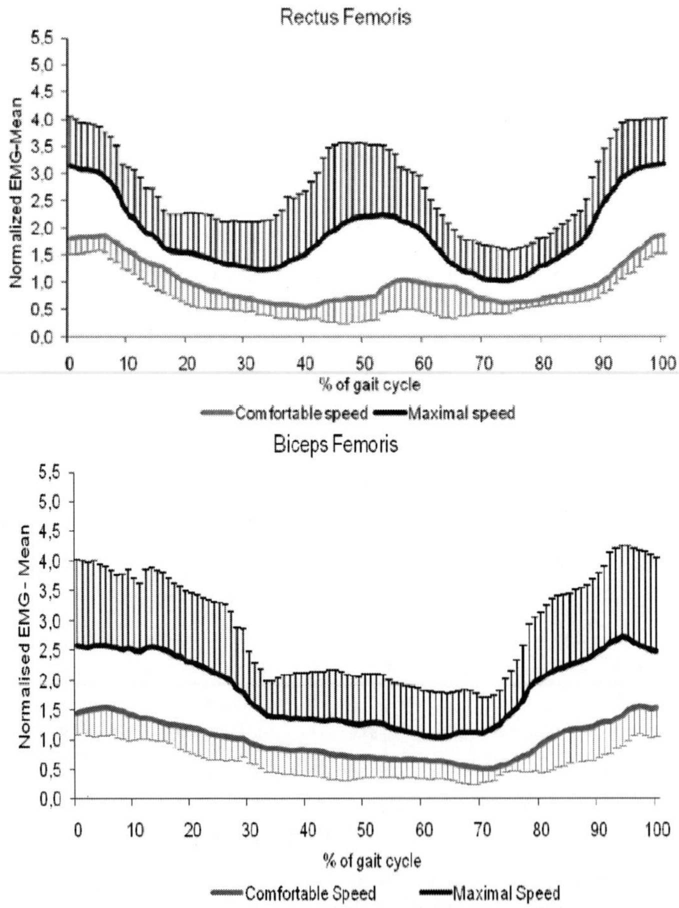

Figure 1. (Continued).

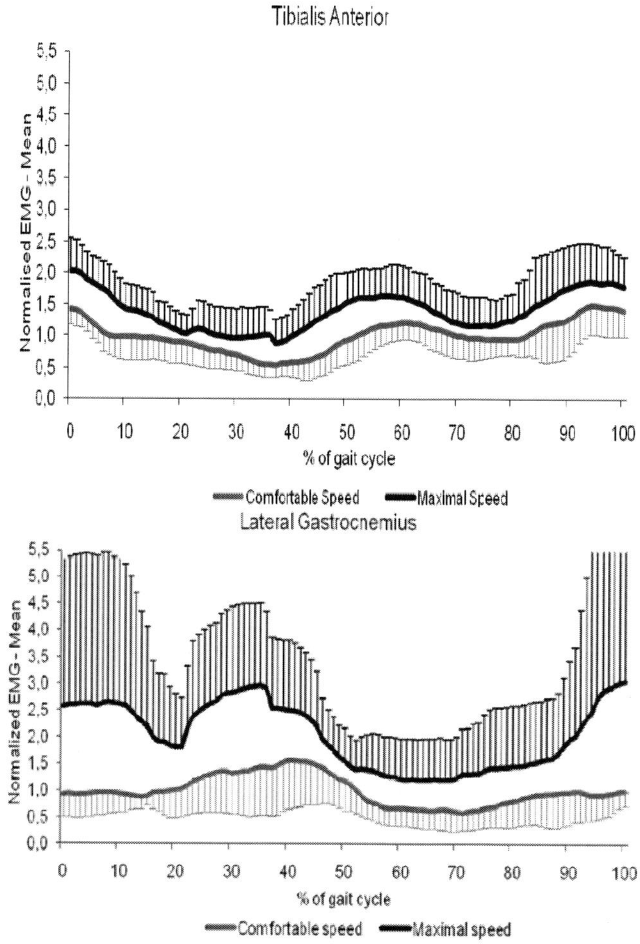

Figure 1. Electromyographic activity (means ±SD) normalized by the mean dynamic method during one complete gait cycle of the paretic lower limb muscles, both at comfortable and maximal speeds.

The lateral gastrocnemius demonstrated distinct patterns at each speed. At the comfortable speed, monophasic patterns of EMG activity were observed from mid-stance (~25%) to the pre-swing (55%).

The highest EMG values were seen in the middle of the terminal stance. At the maximal speed, biphasic patterns were observed: One period began at the terminal swing (~85%) and continued until mid-stance (~20%), and the second period was from around 25% to 55%. of stance. Since this period was common for both speeds, it was thus, selected for analyses.

Comparisons between the Comfortable and Maximal Walking Speeds Considering the Methods of Normalization

The magnitudes of the EMG activity at maximal walking speeds were always greater than those at comfortable speeds for both methods of normalization (Figure 3). For the mean method, the ratios provided in Table 1, ranged from 32 to 126%, greater at the maximal speed. Corresponding values for the peak method ranged from 34 to 122%.

For all statistical analyses, the ANOVAs revealed interaction effects between walking speeds and the methods of normalization ($9.02<F<31.24; 0.001<p<0.016$), indicating that the normalization method had greater effects on the mean data at the maximal speed with the steepest decreasing slope (Figure 3).

Consequently, for most muscles over the analyzed periods of the gait cycles, the greatest differences between speeds were observed for the data normalized by the mean method (Figure 3).

As given in Table 1, the ratios computed from the mean values reported in Figure 3, revealed that at the comfortable and maximal walking speeds, the values of the mean method of normalization were respectively 64 to 100% and 67 to 103% greater than the values obtained by the peak method.

Table 1. Mean magnitudes of the electromyographic activity ratios (%) between each method of normalization at comfortable and maximal walking speeds and between walking speeds normalized by the peak and mean dynamic methods.

Muscle	Gait Cycle	Comfortable: Mean to peak	Maximal: Mean to peak	Peak method Maximal to comfortable	Mean method Maximal to comfortable
RF	0 to 20%	100.00	102.61	57.53	59.59
	35 to 70%	100.00	103.30	121.95	125.61
	80 to 100%	98.31	101.68	101.69	105.13
BF	0 to 35%	75.71	74.80	81.43	80.49
	75 to 100%	82.81	81.60	95.31	94.02
TA	0 to 15%	64.18	67.35	46.27	49.09
	40 to 70%	66.10	68.24	44.07	45.92
	80 to 100%	74.32	71.72	33.78	31.78
LG	25 to 55%	116.39	109.01	81.97	75.76

RF: Rectus femoris; BF: Biceps femoris; TA: Tibialis anterior; LG: Lateral gastrocnemius.

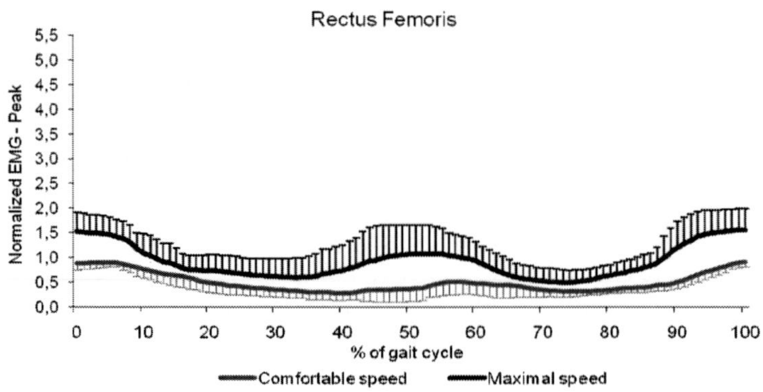

Figure 2. (Continued).

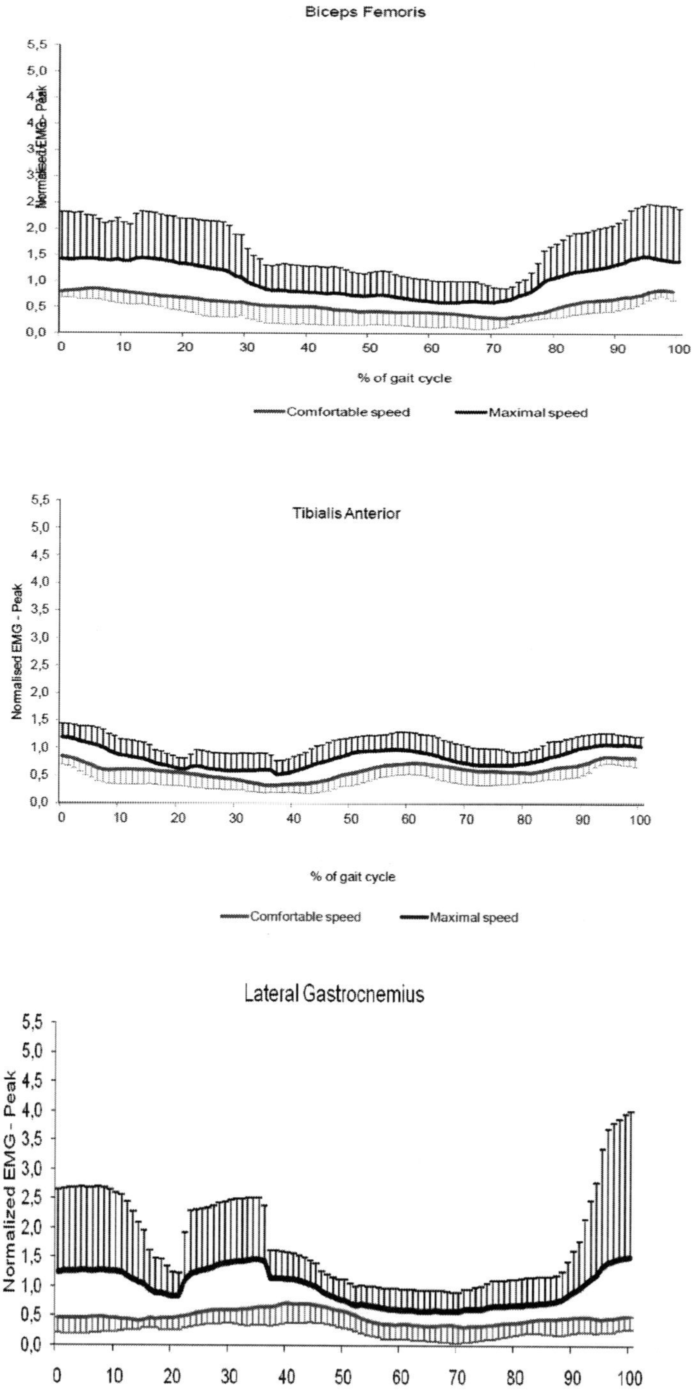

Figure 2. Electromyographic activity (means ±SD) normalized by the peak dynamic method during one complete gait cycle of the paretic lower limb muscles, both at comfortable and maximal speeds.

Intra- and Inter-Subject Variability of the EMG Signal Amplitudes

Table 2 shows the range of the coefficients of variation related to the intra-subject variability at both walking speeds and normalization methods.

For both speeds and methods of normalization, the maximal values were lower than 20%, which indicated that the intra-subject variability was low.

As shown in Figures 1 and 2, differences existed regarding the inter-subject variability of the data obtained by the two normalization methods, with greater standard deviation values generally associated with the mean method.

Observations of the coefficients of variation (Table 3) did not reveal consistent effects of the method on the inter-subject relative variability, except for the rectus femoris, which demonstrated no method effects, since for all analysed gait periods, the coefficient of variation values, obtained by both normalization methods, were lower than 10%.

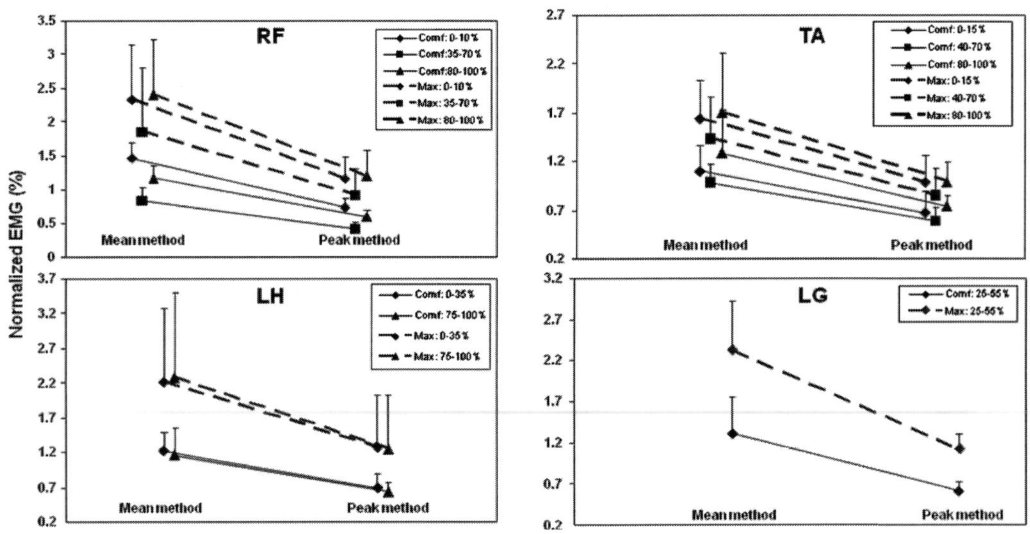

RF: Rectus Femoris; BF: Biceps Femoris; TA: Tibialis Anterior; LG: Lateral Gastrocnemius; Comf: Comfortable speed; Max: Maximal speed.

Figure 3. Mean EMG (±SD) computed over specific periods normalized by both methods at comfortable and maximal speeds.

Observations of the standard deviations (Figure 3) and the coefficients of variation (Table 3) showed that for most muscles over the analyzed periods of the gait cycle, the inter-subject variability of the EMG values at maximal speeds was greater than those obtained at comfortable walking speeds, independent of the method of normalization.

Table 2. Range of intra-subject variability (coefficients of variation, %) of the electromyographic activity at both speeds and normalization methods

Muscle	Gait cycle	Mean method		Peak method	
		Comfortable speed	Maximal speed	Comfortable speed	Maximal speed
RF	0 to 20%	3.23-11.20	3.24-11.43	3.02-16.66	3.73-12.53
	35 to 70%	2.31-19.74	3.85-18.80	6.13-12.14	4.83-19.10
	80 to 100%	5.83-13.70	2.87-13.98	4.50-14.05	3.11-13.29
BF	0 to 35%	0.17-9.17	2.34-19.23	0.40-8.63	1.78-13.55
	75 to 100%	3.63-13.77	3.36-17.30	4.58-14.72	3.15-15.20
TA	0 to 15%	1.27-15.37	1.57-13.83	2.67-11.76	2.42-14.34
	40 to 70%	3.50-8.27	2.44-13.88	3.87-11.62	2.47-19.37
	80 to 100%	4.20-12.80	0.63-10.60	2.34-13.79	1.41-15.74
LG	25 to 55%	4.73-18.07	1.45-13.57	5.76-13.57	3.08-16.44

RF: Rectus femoris; BF: Biceps femoris; TA: Tibialis anterior; LG: Lateral gastrocnemius.

Table 3. Inter-subject variability (coefficients of variation, %) of the electomyographic activity at both speeds and normalization methods

Muscle	Gait cycle	Mean method		Peak method	
		Comfortable speed	Maximal speed	Comfortable speed	Maximal Speed
RF	0 to 20%	15.07	34.76	17.81	28.70
	35 to 70%	24.39	50.81	24.39	43.96
	80 to 100%	14.53	34.17	15.25	32.77
BF	0 to 35%	20.33	47.75	28.57	59.84
	75 to 100%	33.33	54.19	20.31	60.80
TA	0 to 15%	23.64	23.78	32.84	28.57
	40 to 70%	19.39	30.07	23.73	32.94
	80 to 100%	34.11	35.88	14.86	20.20
LG	25 to 55%	40.15	36.64	34.43	45.95

RF: Rectus femoris; BF: Biceps femoris; TA: Tibialis anterior; LG: Lateral gastrocnemius.

Discussion

The overall aim of this chapter was to compare the magnitudes of the EMG signals of the paretic lower limb muscles of stroke subjects walking at comfortable and maximal walking speeds with two forms of normalization, the mean and the peak dynamic methods. The stroke participants had lower comfortable and maximal walking, speeds, compared to values reported for healthy subjects. As reported by Shiavi *et al.* (1987), able-bodied individuals showed a mean comfortable walking speed of 1.44 and maximum of 1.81 m/s. For the present stroke subjects, corresponding values were 0.69 and 1.19, which represented a mean reduction of 52.1 and 34.5%, respectively. Based upon the classification of walking handicaps in a stroke population by Perry *et al.* (1995), the participants fell within the category of "community-walkers" showing full independence in all home and community activities with low risks of falling. The present findings indicated that the method of normalization and the walking speeds modified the EMG activity on the paretic lower limb muscles. The patterns of the peak and the mean methods were differently affected by the walking speeds, since interactions between the walking speeds and normalization methods were observed for all periods of activities for all analyzed muscles.

Pattern Characteristics of EMG Activity

The patterns of the EMG activity were quite similar between the methods of normalization. The periods of gait cycles selected for analyses, which were related to the most important EMG levels of the averaged profiles, were almost equivalent to those chosen by Winter (1991) as being the most important peak activity levels observed during gait of healthy subjects. However, some periods of the most relevant EMG levels of the stroke subjects were slightly longer than those described by Winter (1991), probably due to the fact that they walk slower than healthy subjects. As pointed out by den Otter *et al.* (2004), the amplitude of muscular activity increases with walking speed, due to the need for larger muscular force output. This is because the main role of the muscles in the control of walking speed is to accelerate and decelerate forces of body segments to allow safe forward progression (Winter, 1991). However, since visual inspection was used to determine the EMG onsets and offsets, is is possible that the differences could be partially attributed to the subjectivity of the method itself.

Individual analyses of the EMG activity of each muscle showed that for the rectus femoris and tibialis anterior muscles, the biphasic patterns of EMG activity were quite similar to those of healthy subjects at both walking speeds. As Winter (1991) described, for the rectus femoris, a peak of EMG activity was observed from the end to the beginning of the gait cycle, during weight acceptance phase and after the toe-off to pull the swinging limb forward. For the tibialis anterior, a peak in activity at the beginning of the gait cycle was observed, which corresponded to force generation in opposition to the plantar flexor ground reaction forces. A second important peak in the activity of the tibialis anterior was observed at the end of the stance and during the swing phases, which corresponded to the generation of force for foot clearance. In addition, over all of the analyzed muscles, the tibialis anterior showed the most consistent patterns between the comfortable and maximal walking speeds. For the biceps femoris, a peak in the EMG activity was also observed at the end and beginning of the gait cycle to prepare for weight acceptance.

Finally, for the lateral gastrocnemius, the monophasic patterns observed during comfortable walking speeds changed to biphasic ones at maximal speeds. A new period of EMG activity began at the terminal swing and continued until mid-stance. The period which was similar at both walking speeds was observed during the mid- and late-stance, which was related to the active plantar flexion of the foot and the generation of the most important impulses of energy (Winter,1991). The new burst of EMG activity observed for this muscle from the terminal swing until mid-stance at maximal speeds might be related to the biomechanical demands associated to increases in walking speed (Shiavi *et al.*, 1987) and also to the spasticity of the plantar flexors. The lateral gastrocnemius can act both at the knee and ankle joints and during weight acceptance. The amount of energy absorption at the ankle and knee joints increases at higher walking speeds (Teixeira-Salmela *et al.*, 2008), which could explain the new period of EMG activity observed in this muscle from the terminal swing to mid-stance. In addition, it is important to point out that variance in the EMG signal at maximal speeds also seemed to increase during this period. Considering that this new burst of EMG activity could be related to the biomechanical demands associated with increases in walking speed (Shiavi *et al.*, 1987) and also to the spasticity of the plantar flexors, more motor units need to be recruited. Since the muscles of the paretic lower limb of subjects with stroke demonstrated decreased capacities to activate motor units, as well as reduced numbers of functioning motor units and the motor unit firing rates (Carr and Shepherd, 1998; McComas *et al.*, 1973), greater variability in the EMG signal is observed when more motor units were recruited (Nandedkar, 2002; Grosse *et al.*, 2002).

These results were also, in general, similar to those reported by Shiavi *et al.* (1987), who described the EMG activity pattern characteristics of the lower limb muscles at different walking speeds (free, fast, slow, and very slow) with healthy subjects. The rectus femoris and tibialis anterior muscles showed biphasic patterns for all speeds, and a second distinct period in EMG activity of the gastrocnemius was developed at fast speeds during the swing-to-stance transition. Furthermore, the tibialis anterior had the most consistent patterns across all walking speeds (Shiavi *et al.*, 1987). The EMG pattern characteristics obtained by the two methods of normalization were similar although the magnitudes of the EMG signals varied.

Despite the similarities in the EMG pattern characteristics between the two methods of normalization, in general, the greatest values in the magnitudes of EMG activity were observed for the data normalized by the mean dynamic method and the inter-subject variability was greater at maximal walking speeds. It is important to point out that the analyzed gait trials demonstrated low intra-subject variability, since all of the coefficient of variation values were lower than 20% (Burden *et al.*, 2003; Portney and Watkins, 2000) at both speeds and normalization methods.

Methods of Normalization

An important issue related to EMG analyses is associated with the method of normalization of the EMG signals (Turker, 1993; Yang and Winter, 1984). The most common employed method is the maximum voluntary isometric contraction (MVIC) (Turker, 1993), however, important limitations are associated with this method. The first one is that the MVIC relies upon a voluntary component, which is even further complicated when the data are collected from subjects with pain and/or muscular coordination problems (Cram *et al.*, 1998), as observed in stroke subjects (Carr and Shepherd, 1998; McComas *et al.*, 1973). Another limitation refers to the values used to normalize the EMG data, which are obtained from a specific situation different from the activity of interest (i.e., gait), besides being time consuming (Cram *et al.*, 1998). Finally, the MVIC method showed the highest values of inter-subject variability in previous studies which compared different methods of normalization of the EMG signals of the lower limb muscles during gait (Burden *et al.*, 2003; Yang and Winter, 1984). As pointed out by Yang and Winter (1984), the normalization of EMG activity of the lower limb muscles during gait, with either the peak or the mean dynamic methods, drastically reduced inter-subject variability and increased the sensitivity of surface EMGs as diagnostic tools for gait analyses.

Considering that the main problem in reporting on EMG activity of lower limb muscles of stroke subjects is the inter-individual variability (Den Otter *et al.*, 2007; Olney and Richards, 1996), only the two methods that have shown the lowest variation values (Burden *et al.*, 2003; Yang and Winter, 1984) were compared.

These methods have also the advantage that the normalized values are derived from walking trials (Yang and Winter, 1984). Based on the observed standard deviation values, the peak method showed the lowest variability for all muscles across all intervals of the analyzed gait cycle. However, analyses of the coefficients of variation, which account for relative differences in the magnitude of the means, revealed that the variability of the data was not homogeneous according to the normalization method.

Except for the rectus femoris which showed similar values, the inter-subject variability of the EMGs on the paretic lower limb at different walking speeds and/or at different intervals of the gait cycle, varied in a non-systematic way with one method which provided lower values of inter-subject variability than the other. These observations leave future studies uncertain regarding which method to employ and call for other studies.

Similar results were reported by Shiavi *et al.* (1987), who investigated the inter-subject variability of the EMG data of the lower limb muscles of healthy subjects at comfortable walking speeds normalized by the mean and peak dynamic methods. For the rectus femoris, the peak method showed the lowest coefficient of variation values at both gait speeds.

On the other hand, for the gastrocnemius muscles, the mean method showed the lowest variability values at both gait speeds. As previously stated, amongst the four methods of normalization which have been most investigated, the mean and the peak dynamic methods have been shown to provide lower values of inter-individual variability (Burden *et al.*, 2003; Yang and Winter, 1984). Based upon the present results and on those reported by Shiavi *et al.* (1987), when comparisons between the normalization methods were carried out, the peak appeared to be the most appropriate to reduce inter-subject variability of the EMG activity of the rectus femoris, whereas the mean demonstrated to be most appropriate to reduce inter-subject variability of the gastrocnemius muscles during gait, for healthy and stroke subjects, at both comfortable and maximal walking speeds. For the other muscles, it is recommended to perform initial analyses regarding the best method to reduce inter-subject variability.

In agreement with previous studies which compared EMG activities during gait performance of healthy subjects normalized by these two methods, the present results clearly showed that the mean method produced the highest values of EMG activity at both walking speeds. This may be explained by the fact that for this method, lower values were used to normalize the EMG signals compared to the peak method, resulting in the greatest ratio values (Cram *et al.*, 1998).

Interaction Effects between Walking Speeds and Methods of Normalization

Interactions were found between walking speeds and the methods of normalization for all the assessed gait periods. The differences in EMG activity between comfortable and maximal walking speeds were dependent on the method of normalization.

Therefore, if the aim of a given study is to compare the magnitudes of EMG activity between comfortable and maximal walking speeds, different results would be found depending on the normalization method.

Burden *et al.* (2003) compared four different methods of normalizing EMG signals recorded during the gait of healthy subjects on a treadmill at their normal walking speeds. They also reported similar patterns of muscular activity between the mean and the peak methods.

However, comparisons of the magnitudes of EMG activity were performed only for the isometric and isokinetic maximal voluntary contraction methods of normalization, only in a descriptive manner. The large mean percentage differences between these normalization methods observed by Burden *et al.* (2003) ranged from 21 to 33%.

Since no previous studies were found regarding comparisons of the magnitudes of EMG activity normalized by the employed present methods, it was not possible to conclude that these interactions were only observed for the muscles of the paretic lower limb of stroke subjects.

Therefore, future studies aimed at comparing EMG data during different conditions (walking speeds, pre-post interventions, gait with and without assistive devices) and/or groups, should perform initial analyses of the EMG data considering the various methods of normalization before reporting their main results. This statement must be taken into consideration when the analyses are related to the EMG activity of the paretic lower limb muscles of stroke subjects during gait at maximal speeds. As pointed out, the method of normalization can potentially alter the final results.

EMG Activity at Comfortable and Maximal Walking Speeds

Subjects with a history of stroke are able to increase their walking speeds above their comfortable levels (Bohannon, 1992). The present findings revealed that these subjects were also able to increase the EMG activity of the muscles of the paretic lower limb at maximal walking speeds above the levels observed during comfortable speeds. For all evaluated muscles, the EMG activity was always greater at maximal walking speeds for both methods of normalization.

These findings were similar to those reported by Hesse *et al.* (2001), who investigated the relationships between treadmill speeds and lower limb muscular activity in ambulatory hemiparetic subjects.

They reported positive and significant correlations between these variables (Hesse *et al.*, 2001). Greater walking speeds also increased activation of the paretic lower limb muscles. Similar results were also reported in studies with healthy subjects ((Den Otter *et al.*, 2004; Murray *et al.*, 1984), but the differences in the magnitudes of the EMG activity levels between speeds were considerably lower than those presently found.

Faster walking speeds require greater acceleration and deceleration muscular forces and, thus, are reflected by greater EMG levels. Milot *et al.* (2007) evaluated the paretic lower limb muscles of chronic hemiparetic subjects at comfortable and maximal walking speeds.

They investigated the muscular utilization ratio, an outcome which integrates both muscular strength and gait parameters within the concept of levels of effort, and found that the peak muscular utilization ratios increased with walking speeds.

Besides the greater values of magnitude of the EMG activity at maximal walking speeds, the periods were more clearly determined and the timing periods occurred earlier in the relative stride durations at maximal walking speeds. These results were also supported by Shiavi *et al.* (1987), who described the EMG activity patterns of the lower limb muscles at different walking speeds for healthy subjects.

Conclusion

Increases in EMG activity with faster walking speeds were associated with more variable patterns of muscular activation. For most muscles and intervals of the analyzed gait cycles, the maximal walking speeds showed the greatest variability values for both methods of normalization.

However, previous studies which compared the EMG activity of the lower limb muscles of healthy subjects at different walking speeds reported that, in general, the variability of the EMG signals decreased as speed increased. In stroke subjects, greater variability in the EMG signals of the paretic lower limb muscles may be associated with the utilization of different muscular strategies to increase speed .

The methods of normalization and the walking speeds modified the magnitudes of EMG activity of the paretic lower limb muscles of stroke subjects and the effects of the methods of normalization were greater at maximal walking speeds. The intra-subject variability was lower for both speeds and normalization methods.

However, the inter-subject variability showed higher values, which were not consistently modified by the method of normalization for the analyzed muscles, except for the rectus femoris. Therefore, it is recommended to perform initial analyses of the EMG data, before choosing the best normalization method to reduce inter-subject variability. These results should be considered when the impacts of locomotor interventions on EMG values with stroke subjects are evaluated.

Acknowledgments

The authors are thankful to the Canadian Institute for Health Research (CIHR) for funding the Multidisciplinary Team on Locomotor Rehabilitation after spinal cord Injury and Stroke. CDCM Faria held a scholarship from the Brazilian Government Agency (CAPES); Graduate Student's Exchange Program (Government of Canada), and a student dissertation award from International Society of Biomechanics. MH Milot holds a scholarship from the CIHR. LF Teixeira-Salmela has support from the Brazilian Government Funding Agencies (CAPES, CNPq, and FAPEMIG). S Nadeau has a senior scientist grant from Fonds de la Recherche en Santé du Québec.

References

Berg, K.; Wood-Dauphinée, S.; Williams, J. I. The Balance Scale: Reliability assessment with elderly residents and patients with an acute stroke. *Scandinavia Journal Rehabilitation Medicine,* 1995 27 (1), 27-36.

Bohannon, R. W. Walking after stroke: Comfortable versus maximum safe speed. *International Journal of Rehabilitation Research,* 1992 15 (3), 246-248.

Bohannon, R. W.; Andrews, A. W.; Smith, B. M. Rehabilitation goals of patients with hemiplegia. *International Journal of Rehabilitation Research,* 1988 11 (2), 181-183.

Burden, A. M.; Trew, M; Baltzopoulos, V. Normalisation of gait EMGs: A re-examination. *Journal of Electromyography and Kinesiology,* 2003 13 (6), 519-532.

Carr, J.; Shepherd, R. *Stroke. Neurological Rehabilitation: Optimizing Motor Performance.* Oxford: Butterworth – Heinemann; 1998.

Cram, J. R.; Kasman, G. S.; Holts, J. *Introduction to surface electromyography.* Maryland: Aspen Publishers; 1998.

Cohen, J. J.; Sveen, J. D.; Walker, J. M.; Brummel-Smith, K. Establishing criteria for community ambulation. *Topics in Geriatrics Rehabilitation,* 1987 3 (1), 71-77.

Den Otter, A. R.; Geurts, A. C. H.; Mulder, T.; Duysens J. Speed related changes in muscle activity from normal to very slow walking speeds. *Gait and Posture,* 2004 19 (3), 270-278.

Den Otter, A. R.; Geurts, A. C. H.; Mulder, T. H.; Duysens, J. Abnormalities in the temporal patterning of lower extremity muscle activity in hemiparetic gait. *Gait and Posture,* 2007 25 (3), 342-352.

Engardt, M.; Knutsson, E.; Jonsson, M.; Sternhag, M. Dynamic muscle strength training in stroke patients: Effects on knee extension torque, electromyographic activity, and motor function. *Archives of Physical Medicine and Rehabilitation,* 1995 76 (5), 419-425.

Geyh, S.; Cieza, A.; Schouten, J.; Dickson, H.; Frommelt, P.; Omar, Z.; Kostanjsek, N.; Ring, H.; Stucki, G. ICF Core Sets for stroke. *Journal of Rehabilitaion Medicine,* 2004 44 (Suppl.), 135-141.

Gowland, C.; Stratford, P.; Ward, M.; Moreland, J.; Torresin, W.; Van Hullenaars, S.; Sanford, J.; Barreca, S.; Vanspall, B.; Plews, N. Measuring physical impairment and disability with the Chedoke-McMaster Stroke Assessment. *Stroke.* 1993 24 (1), 58-63.

Grosse, P.; Cassidy, M. J.; Brown, P. EEG-EMG, MEG-EMG and EMG-EMG frequency analysis: Physiological principles and clinical applications. *Clinical Neurophysiology,* 2002 113 (10), 1523-1531.

Hesse, S.; Werner, C.; Paul, T.; Bardeleben, A.; Chaler, J. Influence of walking speed on lower limb muscle activity and energy consumption during treadmil walking of hemiparetic patients. *Archives of Physical Medicine and Rehabilitation,* 2001, 82 (11), 1547-1550.

Jorgensen, H; Nakayama, H; Raaschou, H; Olsen, T. Recovery of walking function in stroke patients: The Compenhagen study. *Archives of Physical Medicine and Rehabilitation.* 1995 76 (1), 27-32.

McComas, A. J.; Sica, R. E. P.; Upton, A. R. M; Aguilera, N. Functional changes in motoneurones of hemiparetic patients. Journal of Neurology, Neurosurgery and Psychiatry, 1973 36 (2), 183-193.

Milot, M. H.; Nadeau, S.; Gravel, D. Muscular utilization of the plantarflexors, hip flexors and extensors in persons with hemiparesis walking at self-selected and maximal speeds. *Journal of Electromyography and Kinesiology.* 2007 17 (2),184-193.

Murray, M. P. ; Mollinger, L. A.; Gardner, G. M.; Sepic, S. B. Kinematic and EMG patterns during slow, free, and fast walking. *Journal of Orthopaedic Research,* 1984 2 (3), 272-280.

Nadeau, S; Arsenault, A. B.; Gravel, D; Bourbonnais, D. Analysis of the clinical factors determining natural and maximal gait speeds in adults with a stroke. *Archives of Physical Medicine and Rehabilitation.* 1999, 78 (2), 123-130.

Nandedkar, S. D. Models and simulations in electromyography. *Muscle and Nerve,* 2002 S11, S46-S54.

Olney, S. J.; Griffin, M. P.; McBride, I. D. Temporal, kinematic, and kinetic variables related to gait speed in subjects with hemiplegia: A regression approach. *Physical Therapy.* 1994, 74 (9), 872-885.

Olney, S. J.; Richards, C. Hemiparetic gait following stroke. Part I: Characteristics. *Gait and Posture.* 1996 4 (2), 136-148.

Perry, J; Garrett, M; Gronley, J. K.; Mulroy, S. J. Classification of walking handicap in the stroke population. *Stroke.* 1995 26 (6), 982-989.

Portney, L. G.; Watkins, M. P. *Foundations of Clinical Research: Applications to Practice.* 2nd Edition. Upper Saddle River, New Jersey: Prentice-Hall Health; 2000.

Salbach, N. M.; Mayo, N. E.; Higgins, J; Ahmed, S; Finch, L. E.; Richards, C. L. Responsiveness and predictability of gait speed and other disability measures in acute stroke. *Archives of Physical Medicine and Rehabilitation,* 2001 82 (9), 1204-1212.

Shiavi, R.; Bugle, H. J.; Limbird, T. Electromyographic gait assessment, part 1: Adult EMG profiles and walkin speed. *Journal of Rehabilitation Research and Development* ,1987 24 (2), 13-23.

Teixeira-Salmela, L. F.; Nadeau, S; McBride, I; Olney, S. J. Effects of muscle strengthening and physical conditioning training on temporal, kinematic and kinetic variables during gait in chronic stroke survivors. *Journal of Rehabilitation Medicine*, 2001 33 (2), 53-60.

Teixeira-Salmela, L. F.; Nadeau, S; Milot, M. H.; Gravel, D.; Requião, L. F. Effects of cadence on energy generation and absorption at lower extremity joints during gait. *Clinical Biomechanics*, 2008 23(6), 769-778.

Turker, K. S. Electromyography: Some methodological problems. *Physical Therapy*, 1993 73 (10), 698-710.

Wade, D. T.; Wood, V. A.; Heller, A; Maggs, J; Langton, R. Walking after stroke: Measurement and recovery over the first 3 months. *Scandinavian Journal of Rehabilitation Medicine*, 1987 19 (1), 25-30.

Winter, D. A. *The biomechanics and motor control of human gait: Normal, elderly, and pathological.* 2nd Edition. Waterloo: University of Waterloo Press; 1991.

Yang, J. F.; Winter, D. A. Electromyographic amplitude normalization methods: Improving their sensitivity as diagnostic tools in gait analysis.*Archives of Physical Medicine and Rehabilitation,* 1984 65 (9), 517-521.

In: Electromyography
Editor: Hiroki Takada
ISBN: 978-1- 62081-717-9

Chapter XI

Two Types of Skeletal Muscle: Power Type and Speed Type

Koshin Mihashi
Graduate School of Mathematics, Nagoya University,
Chikusa-ku, Japan

Abstract

The motion and power of muscle tissue vary greatly among higher and lower animals depending on the condition of the environment in which they live. To provide an example, the motility characteristics of muscle tissues of frogs and turtles are compared in this chapter.

Introduction

Biochemical processes control dynamic motion in muscle tissue. First, in the excitation-contraction coupling machinery of muscles, calcium (Ca^{2+}) allows the interaction of contractile proteins (actin and myosin) to develop force. This complex process (Enoka, 2008) is known as the cross-bridge theory of muscle contraction and is described in detail elsewhere (Huxley, 1957, 2000). Second, the chemical energy of ATP is converted to mechanical force to shorten muscle through the enzymatic reaction of ATPase. In this chapter, we focus on the latter process.

Frog and Turtle Muscles

The reaction sites of ATPase are aligned regularly between 2 kinds of filaments, the myosin thick filament and the F-actin thin filament. As the ATPase reaction proceeds on myosin sites, myosin filaments pull on the F-actin filaments. Owing to this unidirectional movement of the 2 filaments, the ATP energy conversion of muscle works very efficiently (as high as 0.8 energy efficiency in turtle muscle). As the efficiency varies depending on the conditions, a large variety of motions are endowed among members of the animal kingdom. A typical comparison is given in Figure 1 between frog and turtle muscles. When a 10% load is applied to frog and turtle muscle tissues, the shortening speed of frog muscle decreases to about 70%, while that of turtle muscle goes down to 40%. One may consider that frog muscle is tougher (or stronger) than the muscle tissue of turtles. However, the work efficiency of frog muscle can be as low as 10%, while turtle muscle maintains more than 20% efficiency. Turtle muscle tissue uses up ATP better; hence, turtles work more economically than frogs.

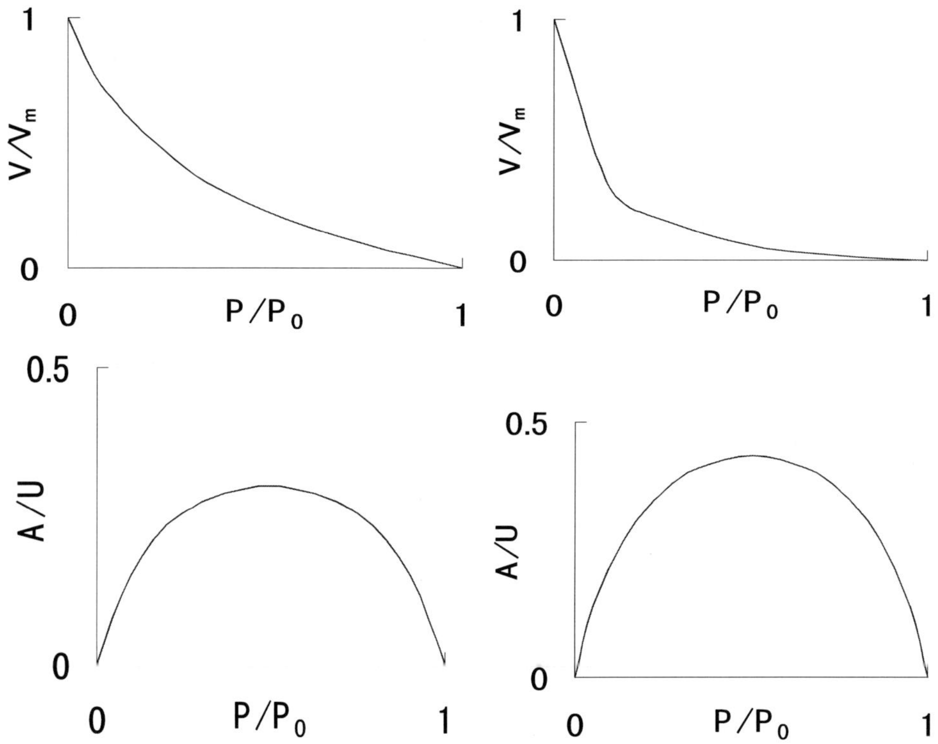

Figure 1. Characteristics of Frog (left) and Turtle (right) Muscle Tissues.

(Top) Contraction velocity, V, as a function of the tension loaded, P (both are relative to the maximum values)

(Bottom) Energy efficiency (A/U) as a function of the tension loaded (both are relative to the maximum values; in the ordinate, A is the rate of work and U is the rate of the total energy consumed)

Table 1. Physical Parameters of Frog and Turtle Muscle Frog Turtle.

(1) Steady-state maximum tension [g/cm^2] 2000 1880

(2) Time for development of

the maximum tension [s] 0.25 4

(3) Maximum shortening speed [μm/s] 1.3 0.3

(4) Time for relaxation [s] 0.063 2.5

(5) Energy efficiency 0.45 0.77

The point is more clearly shown in Table 1 (Woledge, 1968): (1) The steady-state maximum tension, Po, is not largely different between frog and turtle muscles. However, (2) the development of Po in frog tissue occurs rapidly, and (3) the maximum shortening velocity, Vmax, of frog muscle is more than 4 times greater than that of the turtle muscle. Interestingly, (4) the time for relaxation is more than 40 times longer for turtle muscle than for frog muscle. Therefore, it seems likely that the mechanism behind the economical function of turtle tissue is derived from the animal's characteristic "slow life."

Conclusion

In evaluating the various animal muscle tissues, not only the efficiency of energy conversion of individual muscles but also the environmental conditions must be taken into consideration.

References

Enoka, R. *Neuromechanics of Human Movement*, 4th ed. Champaign, IL: Human Kinetics; 2008.

Woledge, R.C. (1968). The energetics of tortoise muscle. *Journal of Physiology*, vol. 197, 685-707.

Huxley, A. F. (1957). Muscle structure and theories of contraction. *Progress in Biophysics and Molecular Biology*, vol.7, 255-318.

Huxley, A. F. (2000). Mechanics and models of the myosin motor. *Philosophical Transactions of the Royal Society*, B355, 433-440.

Index

C

D

J

K

L

M

N

O

P

Q

T

U

V

W

X

Y